Psychiatric Genetics

Review of Psychiatry Series
John M. Oldham, M.D., M.S.
Michelle B. Riba, M.D., M.S.
Series Editors

**Faculty of the Virginia Institute of
Psychiatric and Behavioral Genetics
Departments of Psychiatry and Human Genetics
School of Medicine, Virginia Commonwealth University**

Sam Chen, Ph.D.
Lindon Eaves, Ph.D., D.Sc.
John M. Hettema, M.D., Ph.D.
Kristen C. Jacobson, Ph.D.
Kenneth S. Kendler, M.D.
Hermine H. Maes, Ph.D.
Michael Neale, Ph.D.
Carol A. Prescott, Ph.D.
Brien Riley, Ph.D.
Judy Silberg, Ph.D.

Psychiatric Genetics

EDITED BY

Kenneth S. Kendler, M.D.
Lindon Eaves, Ph.D., D.Sc.

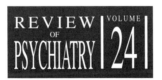

No. 1

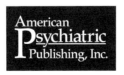

Washington, DC
London, England

Copyright © 2005 American Psychiatric Publishing, Inc.
ALL RIGHTS RESERVED

Manufactured in the United States of America on acid-free paper
09 08 07 06 05   5 4 3 2 1
First Edition

Typeset in Adobe's Palatino

American Psychiatric Publishing, Inc.
1000 Wilson Boulevard
Arlington, VA 22209-3901
www.appi.org

The correct citation for this book is
Kendler KS, Eaves L (editors): *Psychiatric Genetics* (Review of Psychiatry Series, Volume 24, Number 1; Oldham JM and Riba MB, series editors). Washington, DC, American Psychiatric Publishing, 2005

Library of Congress Cataloging-in-Publication Data
Psychiatric genetics / edited by Kenneth S. Kendler and Lindon Eaves.—1st ed.
      p. ; cm. — (Review of psychiatry series ; v. 24, 1)
    Includes bibliographical references and index.
    ISBN 1-58562-228-1 (pbk. : alk. paper)
    1. Mental illness—Genetic aspects
    [DNLM: 1. Mental Disorders—genetics. 2. Mental disorders—
  epidemiology.] I. Kendler, Kenneth S., 1950– II. Eaves, Lindon. III. Series.
    RC455.4.G4P774 2005
    616.89′042—dc22
                                                                        2005002348

British Library Cataloguing in Publication Data
A CIP record is available from the British Library.

Contents

Contributors

Sam Chen, Ph.D.
Department of Psychiatry, Virginia Institute for Psychiatric and Behavioral Genetics, School of Medicine, Virginia Commonwealth University, Richmond, Virginia

Lindon Eaves, Ph.D., D.Sc.
Departments of Human Genetics and Psychiatry. Virginia Institute for Psychiatric and Behavioral Genetics, School of Medicine, Virginia Commonwealth University, Richmond, Virginia

John M. Hettema, M.D., Ph.D.
Department of Psychiatry. Virginia Institute for Psychiatric and Behavioral Genetics, School of Medicine, Virginia Commonwealth University, Richmond, Virginia

Kristen C. Jacobson, Ph.D.
Department of Psychiatry. Virginia Institute for Psychiatric and Behavioral Genetics, School of Medicine, Virginia Commonwealth University, Richmond, Virginia

Kenneth S. Kendler, M.D.
Departments of Psychiatry and Human Genetics, Virginia Institute of Psychiatric and Behavioral Genetics, School of Medicine, Virginia Commonwealth University, Richmond, Virginia

Hermine H. Maes, Ph.D.
Department of Human Genetics, Virginia Institute for Psychiatric and Behavioral Genetics, School of Medicine, Virginia Commonwealth University, Richmond, Virginia

Michael Neale, Ph.D.
Departments of Psychiatry and Human Genetics, Virginia Institute for Psychiatric and Behavioral Genetics, School of Medicine, Virginia Commonwealth University, Richmond, Virginia

John M. Oldham, M.D., M.S.
Professor and Chair, Department of Psychiatry and Behavioral Sciences, Medical University of South Carolina, Charleston, South Carolina

Carol A. Prescott, Ph.D.
Departments of Psychiatry and Psychology, Virginia Institute for Psychiatric and Behavioral Genetics, School of Medicine, Virginia Commonwealth University, Richmond, Virginia

Michelle B. Riba, M.D., M.S.
Clinical Professor and Associate Chair for Education and Academic Affairs, Department of Psychiatry, University of Michigan Medical School, Ann Arbor, Michigan

Brien Riley, Ph.D.
Departments of Psychiatry and Human Genetics, Virginia Institute for Psychiatric and Behavioral Genetics, School of Medicine, Virginia Commonwealth University, Richmond, Virginia

Judy Silberg, Ph.D.
Department of Human Genetics, Virginia Institute for Psychiatric and Behavioral Genetics, School of Medicine, Virginia Commonwealth University, Richmond, Virginia

Introduction to the Review of Psychiatry Series

John M. Oldham, M.D., M.S.
Michelle B. Riba, M.D., M.S.

2005 REVIEW OF PSYCHIATRY SERIES TITLES

- *Psychiatric Genetics*
  EDITED BY KENNETH S. KENDLER, M.D., AND
  LINDON EAVES, PH.D., D.SC.

- *Sleep Disorders and Psychiatry*
  EDITED BY DANIEL J. BUYSSE, M.D.

- *Advances in Treatment of Bipolar Disorder*
  EDITED BY TERENCE A. KETTER, M.D.

- *Mood and Anxiety Disorders During Pregnancy and Postpartum*
  EDITED BY LEE S. COHEN, M.D., AND RUTA M. NONACS, M.D., PH.D.

The Annual Review of Psychiatry has been published for almost a quarter of a century, and 2005 marks the final year of publication of this highly successful series. First published in 1982, the Annual Review was conceived as a single volume highlighting new developments in the field that would be informative and of practical value to mental health practitioners. From the outset, the Annual Review was coordinated with the Annual Meeting of the American Psychiatric Association (APA), so that the material from each year's volume could also be presented in person by the chapter authors at the Annual Meeting. In its early years, the Review was one of a relatively small number of major books regularly published by American Psychiatric Press, Inc. (APPI; now American Psychiatric Publishing, Inc.). Through the subsequent years, however, the demand for new authoritative material led to an exponential growth in the number of new titles published by APPI each year. New published material became more readily available throughout each year, so that the unique function originally provided by the Annual Review was no longer needed.

Times change in many ways. The increased production volume, depth, and diversity of APPI's timely and authoritative material, now rapidly being augmented by electronic publishing, are welcome changes, and it is appropriate that this year's volume of the Annual Review represents the final curtain of the series. We have been privileged to be coeditors of the Annual Review for over a decade, and we are proud to have been a part of this distinguished series.

We hope you will agree that Volume 24 wonderfully lives up to the traditionally high standards of the Annual Review. In *Psychiatric Genetics,* edited by Kendler and Eaves, the fast-breaking and complex world of the genetics of psychiatric disorders is addressed. Following Kendler's clear and insightful introductory overview, Eaves, Chen, Neale, Maes, and Silberg present a careful analysis of the various methodologies used today to study the genetics of complex diseases in human populations. In turn, the book presents the latest findings on the genetics of schizophrenia, by Riley and Kendler; of anxiety disorders, by Hettema; of substance use disorders, by Prescott, Maes, and Kendler; and of antisocial behavior, by Jacobson.

Sleep Disorders and Psychiatry, edited by Buysse, brings us up to date on the sleep disorders from a psychiatric perspective, reviewing critically important clinical conditions that may not always receive the priority they deserve. Following a comprehensive introductory chapter, Buysse then presents, with his colleagues Germain, Moul, and Nofzinger, an authoritative review of the fundamental and pervasive problem of insomnia. Strollo and Davé next review sleep apnea, a potentially life-threatening condition that can also be an unrecognized source of excessive daytime sleepiness and impaired functioning. Black, Nishino, and Brooks present the basics of narcolepsy, along with new findings and treatment recommendations. In two separate chapters, Winkelman then reviews the parasomnias and the particular problem of restless legs syndrome. The book concludes with an extremely important chapter by Zee and Manthena reviewing circadian rhythm sleep disorders.

Advances in Treatment of Bipolar Disorder, edited by Ketter, provides an update on bipolar disorder. Following an introductory overview by Ketter, Sachs, Bowden, Calabrese, Chang, and Rasgon on the advances in the treatment of bipolar disorder, more specific material is presented on the treatment of acute mania, by Ketter, Wang, Nowakowska, Marsh, and Bonner. Sachs then presents a current look at the treatment of acute depression in bipolar patients, followed by a review by Bowden and Singh of the long-term management of bipolar disorder. The problem of rapid cycling is taken up by Muzina, Elhaj, Gajwani, Gao, and Calabrese. Chang, Howe, and Simeonova then discuss the treatment of children and adolescents with bipolar disorder, and the concluding chapter, by Rasgon and Zappert, provides a special focus on women with bipolar disorder.

Mood and Anxiety Disorders During Pregnancy and Postpartum, edited by Cohen and Nonacs, concerns the range of issues of psychiatric relevance related to pregnancy and the postpartum period. Cohen and Nonacs review the course of psychiatric illness during pregnancy, and the postpartum period is covered by Petrillo, Nonacs, Viguera, and Cohen. In this review, the authors focus particularly on depression, bipolar disorder, anxiety disorders, and psychotic disorders. The diagnosis and treatment of mood and anxiety disorders during pregnancy are then discussed in more detail in the subsequent chapter by Nonacs, Cohen, Viguera, and Mogielnicki, followed by a more in-depth look at management of bipolar disorder by Viguera, Cohen, Nonacs, and Baldessarini. Nonacs then presents a comprehensive and important look at the postpartum period, concentrating on mood disorders. This chapter is followed by a discussion of the use of antidepressants and mood-stabilizing medications during breast-feeding, by Ragan, Stowe, and Newport. Overall, this book provides up-to-date information about the management of common psychiatric disorders during gestation and during the critical postpartum period.

Before closing this final version of our annual introductory comments, we would like to thank all of the authors who have contributed so generously to the Annual Review, as well as the editors who preceded us. In addition, we thank the wonderful staff at APPI who have so diligently helped produce a quality product each year, and we would particularly like to thank our two administrative assistants, Liz Bednarowicz and Linda Gacioch, without whom the work could not have been done.

Chapter 1

Introduction

Kenneth S. Kendler, M.D.

Since the mid-1980s, the field of psychiatric genetics has grown in both size and influence. This growth has been paralleled by unprecedented advances in other aspects of human genetics. Unfortunately, as often happens in science, these advances carry with them their own concepts and vocabulary, making the achievements progressively less accessible to the generalist and the clinician.

Our hope in this modest volume for the Review of Psychiatry series is to present, for a general psychiatric audience, some "vignettes" from the exciting world of psychiatric genetics as we see it in the fall of 2004. We quickly realized that with the limited space available to us, a thorough presentation of the field was out of the question. Therefore, rather than trying to cover all the methodological and substantive advances with extreme brevity (and we suspect confusion), we chose a more limited set of subjects that we could explore in more depth. Not surprisingly, the subjects chosen reflect the areas of interest and expertise of the chapter authors, all of whom are on the faculty of the Virginia Institute of Psychiatric and Behavioral Genetics. Some very important areas of research had to be left out. You will not find in this volume discussions of the exciting advances in recent years in genetic studies of major depression, autism, attention-deficit/ hyperactivity disorder, or eating disorders, to name just a few of the neglected areas.

My task in this introductory chapter is twofold. First, I provide a conceptual overview of the field of psychiatric genetics— a brief tour of the major paradigms and methodologies employed in this rapidly growing and changing field. (Many of these issues will be treated in more depth in Chapter 2, "Questions, Models, and Methods in Psychiatric Genetics," by Dr. Eaves and his colleagues.) Second, I orient the reader to the upcoming chapters, describing the main themes that the reader will confront.

The Field of Psychiatric Genetics: The Four Paradigms

Since the early 1980s, several distinct paradigms (Table 1–1) have emerged in psychiatric genetics, from different perspectives, by which investigators have sought to understand the role of genetic factors in the etiology of psychiatric disorders. In this section, I outline these paradigms, review their strengths and weaknesses, and discuss the conceptual issues pertaining to their interrelationships. These questions have been explored in more detail elsewhere (Kendler 2005).

Definitions

Paradigm 1—Basic Genetic Epidemiology

The goal of *basic genetic epidemiology* is to quantify the degree to which individual differences in risk for developing illness result from familial effects (as assessed by a family study) or from genetic factors (as determined by twin or adoption studies). While family, twin, and adoption studies can each be used to address the issues of basic genetic epidemiology, they differ in approach and emphasis. I focus largely on *twin studies* in this discussion because, in addition to being the area of my expertise, such studies have seen the greatest recent growth—with this increased interest driven by the growing number of twin registries (Busjahn 2002) and the introduction of sophisticated analytic tools (Neale et al. 1999).

For twin studies, the task of basic genetic epidemiology is to estimate the proportion of liability in a given population due to genetic differences between individuals (referred to as *heritability*). In this introductory chapter, I refer to "genes" identified by genetic epidemiological methods as *genetic risk factors* to distinguish them from *susceptibility genes* identified by paradigms 3 and 4.

Table 1–1. Four major paradigms of psychiatric genetics

Paradigm	Samples studied	Method of inquiry	Scientific goal(s)
Basic genetic epidemiology	Family, twin, and adoption studies	Statistical	Quantify the degree of familial aggregation and/or heritability
Advanced genetic epidemiology	Family, twin, and adoption studies	Statistical	Explore the nature and mode of action of genetic risk factors
Gene finding	High-density families, trios, case-control samples	Statistical	Determine the genomic location and identity of susceptibility genes
Molecular genetics	Individuals	Biological	Identify critical DNA variants and trace the biological pathways from DNA to disorder

Paradigm 2—Advanced Genetic Epidemiology

Given the demonstration of significant heritability, the goal of *advanced genetic epidemiology* is to explore the nature and mode of action of these genetic risk factors. Some of the many possible questions that can be asked in advanced genetic epidemiology (most of which will be addressed at some point in this book) are as follows (Kendler 1993, 2001):

1. Are the genetic risk factors specific to a given disorder or shared with other disorders?
2. Do the genetic risk factors impact on disease risk similarly in males and females?
3. Do the genetic risk factors moderate the impact of environmental risk factors on disease liability (genetic control of sensitivity to the environment) (Kendler and Eaves 1986)?
4. Do the genetic risk factors impact on disease risk by altering the probability of exposure to environmental risk factors (genetic control of exposure to the environment) (Kendler and Eaves 1986)?
5. Does the action of the risk factors change as a function of the developmental stage of the individual?
6. Do historical experiences moderate the impact of the genetic risk factors so that heritability might differ across historical cohorts?
7. For disorders with multiple stages (i.e., substantial alcohol consumption must precede but does not always lead to alcohol dependence), what is the relationship between the genetic risk factors for these various stages?

In both basic and advanced genetic epidemiological research paradigms, it is critical to emphasize that genetic risk factors are not directly measured. Rather, their existence is inferred from the patterns of resemblance among particular classes of relatives, such as monozygotic versus dizygotic twins or biological parents and their adopted-away offspring.

Paradigm 3—Gene Finding

The goal of *gene-finding* methods is to determine the locations in the genome of genes (or more technically, *loci*) that, when variation occurs, influence liability for developing psychiatric disorders. While molecular methods are used for detecting the genetic variants (or "markers") that are critical to these analyses, gene-finding methods are statistical in nature. By examining the distribution of genetic markers within families or populations, these methods (linkage and/or association) allow us to infer the probability that a locus in the genomic region under investigation contributes to disease liability. A further and more refined goal for paradigm 3 is to clarify the history of the pathogenic variant or variants in the susceptibility gene by determining the background pieces of DNA (termed *haplotypes*) on which these variants are found.

Paradigm 4—Molecular Genetics

The goal of the *molecular genetic* paradigm is to trace the biological mechanisms by which the DNA variant identified using gene-finding methods contributes to the disorder itself. The first task is to identify the change in gene function and/or expression resulting from the identified DNA variant. The subsequent, more difficult task is to trace, using a range of available methods (e.g., molecular, pharmacological, imaging, neuropsychology), the etiological pathway(s) from the DNA variant to the abnormal brain/mind functioning that characterizes the disorder.

Strengths and Limitations

Basic Genetic Epidemiology

Basic genetic epidemiology has the following critical strengths:

1. Permits determination of heritability, which, if convincingly demonstrated, allows us to reject definitively the "radical environmentalist" position that a clustering of illness within families is ipso facto evidence that familial-environmental risk factors are important. Such claims are still commonly made in the psychological, sociological, or epidemiological literature.
2. Allows assessment of the aggregate effects of all genetic risk factors, regardless of their location on the genome or their individual effect size, and therefore provides an overall assessment for a given population of the etiological importance of genetic variation.

3. Provides a foundation, when positive results are obtained, for further work using the methods of advanced genetic epidemiology.

Basic genetic epidemiology has the following critical limitations:

1. Is descriptive in nature and therefore does not provide insight into causal or explanatory pathways. The ultimate goal of science is the elucidation of causal processes. For this purpose, the basic genetic epidemiological paradigm is somewhat unsatisfactory because it is fundamentally descriptive in nature. That is, this method quantifies the importance of genetic risk factors but does not provide insight into causal or explanatory pathways.

2. Draws inferences from estimates of heritability and thus is subject to the limitations of this approach, such as the following:

   - Heritability estimates apply only to populations and not to individuals.
   - In a given population with a particular set of genes, the heritability of a disorder is not immutable and changes when new sources of environmental risk are introduced. Thus, the magnitude of heritability *is not solely a result of the effects of genes.* Rather, it is the ratio of the variance in risk in a population due to genetic differences between the individual and the total variance of risk in that population. Therefore, contrary to common usage, heritability is *not* a characteristic of a disorder or a trait but only of a disorder or trait *in a specific population at a specific time.*
   - The relationship between heritability and feasibility of gene finding is strong only at one extreme; if heritability is zero, gene-finding methods cannot succeed. However, with nonzero heritability estimates, the magnitude of the heritability estimate provides little to no information about the ease of gene finding. Heritability assesses only aggregate genetic effect and is uninformative about the distribution of genetic risk across the genome. It can be easy to find genes

for traits with low heritability if most of that genetic risk is concentrated in one genomic location and/or the genetic effects are particularly strong only in some families. It can be very difficult to localize genetic risk for a disorder with high heritability if the disorder is influenced slightly by variation at many genes widely spread throughout the genome.

- For the estimate of heritability, twin studies rely critically on excess phenotypic resemblance in monozygotic versus dizygotic twins. Nongenetic processes that cause such excess resemblance will bias heritability estimates. Although evidence suggests that such biases are probably not large (Kendler 1993), the observational, nonexperimental nature of genetic epidemiology makes it difficult to rule out such biases definitively.

Advanced Genetic Epidemiology

The most important strength of advanced genetic epidemiological methods is that they move beyond the descriptive approach of paradigm 1 to an exploration of the action of genetic (and environmental) risk factors. Some of these methods can incorporate environmental risk factors or intermediate phenotypes in the analyses. Most importantly, many of these approaches allow us to begin to address questions of causal processes.

The major limitations of advanced genetic epidemiological methods are extensions of those already listed above for the basic methods. Although such advanced methods can begin to address causal issues, they do so by tracing processes between latent statistically defined genetic risk factors. For example, the latent genetic risk factors for major depression and schizophrenia may in part act by influencing the personality trait of neuroticism (Fanous et al. 2002; Kendler et al. 2002) and attentional and executive processes (Cannon et al. 2000; Goldberg et al. 1995), respectively. Since neuroticism and attention are more basic constructs than major depression and schizophrenia, these analyses would constitute a *reductive form* of explanation—that is, one that defines a higher-order complex phenomenon as a manifestation of simpler, more basic processes. However, advanced genetic epidemiology offers only *partial reductive explanations* involving several adjacent levels of a complex causal chain. These causal explanations cannot reach the level of basic genetic/biological processes such as DNA base-pair variation (Sarkar 1998).

Gene Finding

Gene-finding methods have the following critical strengths:

1. Have a basis in well-characterized biological processes. Although gene-finding methods are statistical in nature, the underlying assumptions of these methods are firmly based on the well-characterized biological process of meiosis—that is, genetic recombination and segregation.
2. Yield results that are more specific, informative, and falsifiable than those from basic genetic epidemiology and that are therefore, by most criteria, of greater scientific value (Chalmers 1999).
3. Provide a sound basis for further work within the molecular genetic paradigm. Because these methods are based on sound and well-understood genetic principles, positive results for gene-finding methods present a natural basis for further work using the molecular genetic paradigm.

Gene-finding methods have the following critical limitations:

1. Assess the ratio of genetic to total variance in liability and thus yield evidence that is not independent of environmental risk factors. Like heritability calculations, the statistical methods for gene localization do not solely reflect gene action but rather assess the ratio of genetic to total variance in liability. The evidence for linkage in a family would vary as a function of the potency and frequency of environmental risk factors to which its members were exposed.
2. Do not allow easy identification of a single susceptibility gene. Although gene-finding methods detect susceptibility genes over small regions of the genome, there is no guarantee that the actual susceptibility gene itself can be easily determined. Even with relatively large samples, the size of the "high risk" region detected by linkage analysis can be quite

large, containing dozens to hundreds of possible susceptibility genes (Roberts et al. 1998). In experimental organisms, researchers are seeing single "signals" obtained by gene-finding methods that, on closer examination, actually reflect multiple individual genetic loci.

3. Yield less reliable positive results than do basic genetic epidemiology methods. Whereas basic genetic epidemiology performs *one test* for the presence of genetic risk factors, gene-finding methods involve performing many individual tests to detect susceptibility genes. Because genetic risk factors have been found for nearly all psychiatric and substance abuse disorders examined to date, the hypothesis tested in paradigm 1 (e.g., genetic risk factors exist for disorder X) has a high prior probability. By contrast, the hypothesis tested in gene-finding methods—namely, that a small region of the genome contains a susceptibility gene for disorder X—is much less likely to be true. Statistical theory predicts that positive results from basic genetic epidemiological studies (one test with high a priori probability) will prove much more reliable than positive results from gene-finding methods (many tests with low a priori probabilities). This prediction has been well borne out.

Molecular Genetics

Molecular genetic methods have one overwhelming strength: they raise the possibility of *reductive biological explanations* that would elucidate the causal chain from molecular variation in DNA to the manifestations of psychiatric disorders. Unlike the other three paradigms, the molecular genetic paradigm is not fundamentally statistical in nature but reflects rather the biological reductive model of science that has been frequently successful in biomedicine.

Molecular genetics has one noteworthy weakness: many practical problems stand in the way of clarifying what may be the extraordinarily complex biological pathways from DNA variation to psychiatric disorders. The individual genetic variants that cause classic genetic disorders are usually easy to detect, because they reflect alterations in coding for key amino acids or the destruction of well-defined regulatory sequences. However, the

DNA variants that predispose to complex diseases (including psychiatric disorders) may be more subtle in their action and more difficult to detect. Efforts to understand in basic biological terms even the simplest of behaviors in model organisms have met with substantial difficulties. Molecular genetics also must be concerned about how disease risk arises from interactions between genetically controlled biological processes and environmentally induced changes in brain function.

However, the power of molecular biology and neuroscience is increasing rapidly, so there is reason for guarded optimism that if pathogenic DNA variants are found for psychiatric disorders, they will ultimately make it possible to gain invaluable insights into the etiology of these disorders.

Interrelationships Among Paradigms

Within the field of psychiatric genetics, how should these paradigms interrelate? Positive results from paradigm 1 lead directly to questions posed in paradigm 2. In confirming the statistical signals of gene-finding studies (paradigm 3), it is natural to study the biological changes produced by these genetic variants (paradigm 4). More problematic is the nature of the relationship between paradigms 1 and 2 (hereafter *genetic epidemiology*) and paradigms 3 and 4 (hereafter *gene identification*).

The crux of this problem is the relationship between *genetic risk factors* as defined by genetic epidemiology and *susceptibility genes* as defined by gene identification methods. Put in other terms: Are genetic risk factors simply the statistical signals of susceptibility genes? This question can be framed in more philosophical language as, Do genetic risk factors reduce to susceptibility genes?

This deceptively complex question deserves to be evaluated with great care because it can be addressed on two different levels with divergent answers. On a *theoretical* level, the results of twin and adoption studies, if the studies were properly conducted, should reflect the distal effects of genetic variation coded in DNA. At this theoretical level, therefore, the answer to this question is clear: genetic risk factors are nothing more than signals of susceptibility genes.

However, at a *practical* level, the answer is murky in at least two important ways. First, it can be genuinely debated whether it will ever be possible, regardless of technological advances, to trace in a clear and unambiguous fashion a complete set of causal links from DNA base pair variation to a complex biobehavioral phenomenon such as schizophrenia or major depression.

Second, if genetic risk factors are just manifestations of susceptibility genes, we should be able to use paradigm 3 to confirm the results of paradigm 1. If there is a dispute about whether a twin or adoption study was correct in its conclusion that disorder X is heritable, then we should be able to evaluate these results by linkage and/or association studies. However, although this idea may seem sensible, it is, in practical terms, wrong. If a twin study of disorder X indicated a heritability of 40% and a well-done genome scan showed no regions of significant linkage, it would not be sound to argue, on the basis of the linkage result, that the twin study was in error.

This apparently paradoxical situation is largely due to the blunt power of gene identification methods combined with the possibility that genetic risk factors may reflect the combined signal of many susceptibility genes of small individual effect. With an infinite sample size, genotyping methods without error, and yet to be designed statistical tools, it might *theoretically* be *possible* for gene identification methods to uncover all of the susceptibility genes that form the biological basis for genetic risk factors and to understand how they combine and interact to produce a specific level of disease liability. Whether this will ever be possible is open to debate. If it is possible, we are currently a very long way from that goal.

The practical difficulty of moving from paradigms 1 and 2 to paradigms 3 and 4 leaves a gap in the conceptual framework of psychiatric genetics. It is not yet clear whether we can easily get from genetic risk factors to susceptibility genes. Therefore, genetic epidemiological and gene identification paradigms do not currently relate to one another as do many paradigms in the physical sciences in which results at a more abstract level can be clearly reduced to, and definitively confirmed or refuted by, the application of more basic methods.

Competing Paradigms

Some historical periods in science are marked by competing paradigms (Kuhn 1996). Such an historical/sociological perspective can be usefully applied to the field of psychiatric genetics where two broad camps, that have adopted genetic epidemiology and gene-identification methods as their main paradigm, struggle with each other to attract resources and students. Competition between scientific paradigms most commonly results in one of two outcomes: *replacement* or *integration*. In replacement, one paradigm loses, disappearing from the scientific scene. This was the resolution of the competition between the Ptolemaic and Copernican models for planetary motion. In *integration*, the two paradigms are incorporated into a unified approach. For example, the older paradigm might serve as a useful approximation for the newer paradigm in a limited set of circumstances.

Which of these models best applies to the competing paradigms within psychiatric genetics? While the future is uncertain, a time may come when it is easy and cheap to sequence individual genomes and when, with development of sufficient statistical tools, gene-identification methods will completely replace genetic epidemiology. Instead of having to infer genetic risk factors from patterns of resemblance across relatives as is now done in genetic epidemiological paradigms, it may be possible to measure directly all relevant variants within susceptibility genes and know how to combine this information with relevant environmental exposures to determine individual liability. This will effect a great increase in statistical power because genetic risk could be determined directly and would not need to be inferred by the risk of illness in relatives.

However, such capabilities, if they are achievable, will not be available for a substantial period of time. Therefore, the field of psychiatric genetics would be better served currently by working toward a model of integration. Such a model would require an appreciation of the complementary sources of information obtained by genetic epidemiological and gene-identification approaches. The major advantage of genetic epidemiological methods is that they permit us to assess the magnitude of total genetic influences and then explore how those influences act and interact with various aspects of the internal and external environments. However, most of these questions can also be addressed by means of gene-identification methods, but only at the level of specific genes or genomic regions. Two examples will illustrate this development. Advanced genetic epidemiology has suggested that the genetic risk factors for the personality trait of neuroticism may be correlated but may not be identical in men and women (Eaves et al. 1998; Fanous et al. 2002). A recent linkage study of neuroticism suggested specific genomic locations for these genes that impact differentially in the two sexes (Fullerton et al. 2003). A prior twin study suggested that genetic risk factors for major depression in part act through increasing sensitivity to the depressogenic effects of stressful life events (Kendler et al. 1995). A recent association study has suggested that having a variant in the serotonin transporter gene increases an individual's risk for developing depression after exposure to high levels of stress (Caspi et al. 2003). These two kinds of knowledge (at the aggregate level for all genetic risk factors and at the level of specific susceptibility genes) are by their nature complementary.

However, there are also important questions asked of psychiatric genetics, as in the following examples, that can only be well answered at the level of aggregate risk.

- A large private foundation wants to invest considerable research funds in investigating the etiology of disorder X. In determining how to divide these funds between strategies emphasizing genetic versus environmental risk factors, they turn to psychiatric genetics and ask, "Overall, how important are genetic versus environmental risk factors for disorder X?"
- A committee for DSM-V is having a hard time determining whether syndromes A and B should be placed in the same or different diagnostic categories. They plan to collect data on several diagnostic validators (such as response to treatment and course). However, given prior evidence that both syndromes are heritable, they are particularly hopeful that genetic studies will provide definitive information about how closely related the genetic risk factors are for these two disorders.

- A state legislature is considering a large program to reduce youth access to alcohol, hoping that it will reduce future rates of alcoholism. The legislators know that early onset of alcohol use is associated with later alcoholism, but they turn to psychiatric genetics to help them evaluate whether that link is causal. Does early-onset alcohol use actually cause future alcoholism, or does the association between early onset of alcohol use and later alcoholism result from their both being manifestations of an underlying (partly genetic) liability to deviancy?
- A research team is funded to conduct a large controlled trial of antipsychotic agents in individuals with schizotypal personality disorder. To increase their chances of obtaining positive results, the team members turn to psychiatric genetics to obtain a definition of this disorder that maximizes its genetic relationship to schizophrenia.

In each of these scenarios, the question cannot currently be answered by means of gene-identification methods. Answering these questions requires the ability to assess total genetic risk, and such assessment is currently possible only with genetic epidemiological methods.

The Structure of This Book

In picking the topics for the chapters in this book, we were guided by the following themes. First, the field of psychiatric genetics cannot be appreciated without some conceptual and statistical background. Dr. Eaves and colleagues focus on these issues in Chapter 2, trying to present them in as "user-friendly" a manner as possible. That chapter, longer than the others, presents, in an accessible manner, many of the basic principles of both genetic epidemiology and gene finding, as well as a brief review of DNA itself.

Second, we wanted to present, in some depth, the results for one disorder in which substantial progress has been made in paradigms 3 (gene finding) and 4 (molecular genetics). The choice of schizophrenia was easy to make because progress with these paradigms in this disorder has been substantial in the past several years.

Third, it was important to present results for a more typical and common set of psychiatric disorders for which the bulk of our information comes from paradigms 1 and 2 (basic and advanced genetic epidemiology) and in the study of which we are beginning, using paradigm 3, to make some advances. We chose to present anxiety disorders as particularly illustrative of these sets of issues.

Fourth, major advances have been made (with paradigms 1 and 2) in the study of substance use disorders. Several decades ago the leading paradigm for these syndromes focused on sociological factors and "weakness of character." Now, an increasing number of high-quality genetic epidemiological studies have shown that genetic factors play a large etiological role in these disorders. Furthermore, the genetics of substance use disorders, unlike those of more traditional psychiatric disorders, must consider the inherent conditionality of drug abuse. That is, to develop drug abuse or dependence, you first have to use the substance and typically use it a lot. This raises several questions about the best approach to genetic modeling for these disorders, which we explore in Chapter 5 ("Genetics of Substance Use Disorders").

Fifth, we wanted to explore what has been learned about the genetics of personality disorders. Again, the choice of the externalizing disorder antisocial personality disorder was easy because we have learned much more about this disorder than is known for nearly any other Axis II condition. Furthermore, this choice allowed us, as Dr. Jacobson illustrates in Chapter 6 ("Genetic Influence on the Development of Antisocial Behavior"), to elaborate a further important theme of psychiatric genetics—namely, incorporation of developmental processes in our analyses.

Before we begin, we have to issue a warning. Psychiatric genetics is now a "fact-filled" field. Our struggle in writing this book was to provide accounts that, while thorough and scholarly, are also accessible. To give you the reader a sense of the field, we felt we had to present the relevant data. It would not work just to give a broad "birds-eye" view with a series of sweeping generalizations. So, readers need to be aware: you will be confronting lots of information. Our advice would be to "sit back and relax" as you read this volume. None of the individual bits of data are themselves important. What is important to take away from this book is the broad trends that are emerging in the literatures reviewed, the strengths and limitations of the available methods in providing real insight into the etiology of psychiatric and substance use disorders, and, hopefully, a sense of the excitement of this active field of inquiry. We will have succeeded as authors if these perspectives have been well conveyed.

References

Busjahn A: Twin registers across the globe: what's out there in 2002? (editorial). Twin Research 5:5–6, 2002

Cannon TD, Huttunen MO, Lonnqvist J, et al: The inheritance of neuropsychological dysfunction in twins discordant for schizophrenia. Am J Hum Genet 67:369–382, 2000

Caspi A, Sugden K, Moffitt TE, et al: Influence of life stress on depression: moderation by a polymorphism in the 5-HTT gene. Science 301:386–389, 2003

Chalmers AF: What Is This Thing Called Science? An Assessment of the Nature and Status of Science and Its Methods, 3rd Edition. Indianapolis, IN, Hackett Publishing, 1999

Eaves LJ, Heath AC, Neale JM, et al: Sex differences and non-additivity in the effects of genes on personality. Twin Research 1(3):131–137, 1998

Fanous A, Gardner CO, Prescott CA, et al: Neuroticism, major depression and gender: a population-based twin study. Psychol Med 32:719–728, 2002

Fullerton J, Cubin M, Tiwari H, et al: Linkage analysis of extremely discordant and concordant sibling pairs identifies quantitative-trait loci that influence variation in the human personality trait neuroticism. Am J Hum Genet 72:879–890, 2003

Goldberg TE, Torrey EF, Gold JM, et al: Genetic risk of neuropsychological impairment in schizophrenia: a study of monozygotic twins discordant and concordant for the disorder. Schizophr Res 17:77–84, 1995

Kendler KS: Twin studies of psychiatric illness: current status and future directions. Arch Gen Psychiatry 50:905–915, 1993

Kendler KS: Twin studies of psychiatric illness: an update. Arch Gen Psychiatry 58:1005–1014, 2001

Kendler KS: Psychiatric genetics: a methodologic critique. Am J Psychiatry 2005

Kendler KS, Eaves LJ: Models for the joint effect of genotype and environment on liability to psychiatric illness. Am J Psychiatry 143:279–289, 1986

Kendler KS, Kessler RC, Walters EE, et al: Stressful life events, genetic liability and onset of an episode of major depression in women. Am J Psychiatry 152:833–842, 1995

Kendler KS, Gardner CO, Prescott CA: Toward a comprehensive developmental model for major depression in women. Am J Psychiatry 159:1133–1145, 2002

Kuhn TS: The Structure of Scientific Revolutions, 3rd Edition. Chicago, IL, University of Chicago Press, 1996

Neale MC, Boker SM, Xie G, et al: Mx: Statistical Modeling, 5th Edition. Richmond, VA, Department of Psychiatry, Medical College of Virginia and Virginia Commonwealth University, 1999

Roberts SB, MacLean CJ, Neale MC, et al: Replication of linkage studies of complex traits: an examination of variation in location estimates. Am J Hum Genet 65:876–884, 1999

Sarkar S: Genetics and Reductionism. New York, Cambridge University Press, 1998

Chapter 2

Questions, Models, and Methods in Psychiatric Genetics

Lindon Eaves, Ph.D., D.Sc.
Sam Chen, Ph.D.
Michael Neale, Ph.D.
Hermine H. Maes, Ph.D.
Judy Silberg, Ph.D.

The science of human behavior and its disorders is forged from two seemingly incompatible endeavors. The first seeks to reduce the complexities of behavior to elementary mechanisms that can be manipulated and modified by technological means. This approach seeks the individual genes and processes at the cellular and neurobiological levels out of which behavior is ultimately forged. Enthusiasm for reduction, however, is moderated by the conviction that organisms create their own rules and destinies—that when genes produce brains and people, processes emerge that must be understood and even modified in their own terms. The most skilled treatment of behavioral disorders requires a judicious balance of pharmacology and psychotherapy and implicitly recognizes the intellectual power and clinical significance of both reductionist and holistic approaches.

Some physicians and psychologists may complain that psychiatric genetics is "too reductionist." Cell and molecular biologists sometimes complain that psychiatric genetics is "not reductionist enough." The truth may ultimately yield only to a creative dialogue between these two approaches. Modern psychiatric and behavioral genetics has been fertilized by both. The driving theory of almost all research in behavioral and psychiatric genetics is the conviction that without DNA there is no person, and that we ignore it at our peril. This does not mean that psychiatric geneticists fail to consider the person or the environment; much the reverse. We recognize that *if* genes affect the brain, their effects may pervade every interchange between people and their environment. In short, human behavior cannot be understood apart from the genes.

In this chapter, we outline some of the methods used by researchers as they attempt to uncover the processes that lead to behavioral disorders. The extent of the subject and the diversity of approaches admit only a cursory survey of the principal concepts and methods. We list some of the questions that motivate us and consider some of the models that allow questions to be turned into testable hypotheses. Finally, we illustrate some of the methods that help us test our ideas.

Measuring Variation

Psychiatric genetics aims to explain variation in susceptibility to psychiatric disorders. We often think of diseases as discrete entities, for example, the individual is either "depressed" or "not depressed." Such categories are frequently arbitrary, having been chosen for convenience or for reasons pertaining to the relative costs and benefits of intervention. The decision to characterize someone as "hypertensive" is usually based on whether their diastolic blood pressure exceeds some threshold (e.g., 90 mm Hg). The choice of threshold does not necessarily imply anything fundamental about the underlying causes or biology of hypertension; it merely reflects a current judgment about when medical intervention is likely to be beneficial and cost-effective. Decisions about "where to draw the line" change as medical research obtains better information about the long-term consequences of particular trait levels. As understanding advances, so do the standards of assessment and the criteria for clinical intervention.

Most human differences, such as those in stature or blood pressure, are seldom all or nothing. Height measurements fall into

Proportion

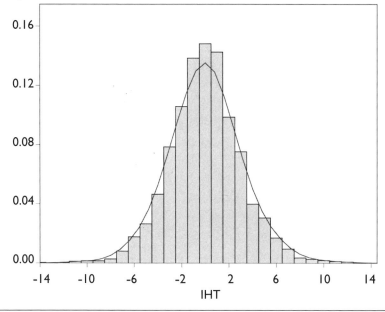

IHT

Figure 2–1. Continuous variation in stature.
Distribution of stature (IHT [height grouped by inches expressed]), represented as inches from mean, is corrected for age and sex.

continuous gradations, with units of measurement limited only by the precision of the instrument. Figure 2–1 illustrates the distribution of stature in a sample from one of our own studies. Subjects are grouped to the nearest inch, but the continuous "normal," or "Gaussian," curve comes very close to describing the relative frequencies of the different trait values.

Susceptibility to psychiatric disorders can be conceived in similar terms. People may differ in their liability to depression much as they differ in stature or blood pressure. The greater a person's liability, the more likely he or she is to express the disorder and to require medical help (Figure 2–2). Sometimes, natural variation in the disease implies that the simple "all or nothing" model is not correct. Psychiatric disorders often show continuous variation in severity, age at onset, number of symptoms, levels of stress, or family history; this suggests that the underlying susceptibility is better conceived as continuously graded, even though,

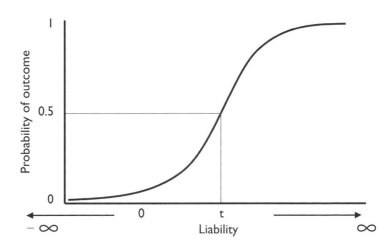

Figure 2–2. Probability of being affected by a disorder as a function of liability.

for the purposes of treatment, a "yes/no" decision has to be made about when intervention is indicated (see Falconer 1965, Chapter 18). The statistical foundation for this work was laid by Karl Pearson (1900), who developed the polychoric correlation to quantify the underlying correlation between relatives for categorical variables. His approach is still widely used today.

Diathesis and Stress: Variation in Risk and Susceptibility

Gregor Mendel (1866/1958), in his *Experiments in Plant Hybridization,* showed that different forms of genes behave mathematically as discrete particles that produce all-or-nothing states. How do discrete particles produce continuous traits like stature or liability to a complex disorder? In 1918, Ronald Fisher, in his classic work on the correlation between relatives on the supposition of Mendelian inheritance, considered what would happen if continuous traits were influenced by more than one gene. Figure 2–3A shows what the distribution of stature would look like if there were just two genes (loci) affecting height, each existing in two equally frequent forms (alleles). One form adds nothing to height, and the other adds one unit. In this case, since each individual samples two alleles (increasing or not) from each of two loci, there would be five distinct height categories corresponding to the five unique combinations of genes ("genotypes") with discrete values of height. Figure 3B shows how even small, random environmental effects can smooth out the distinctions between genetic categories even when the number of genes is very small. In this example, most of the differences are still accounted for by genetic factors, but it is hard to separate the individuals into distinct "genetic" categories. Fisher considered the effects of many more genes. Figure 2–3C shows the distribution of a trait that is affected by 100 genes even in the absence of environment effects. The distribution looks remarkably like that for stature. This recognition that continuous traits might be caused by large numbers of genes, with effects blurred by the environment, led Fisher to formulate his *polygenic theory* of continuous variation. With some minor modifications, Fisher's theory gave a remarkably good account of much of the data that have been gathered for several human measures, including stature, IQ, and personality.

Genes, Environment, and Gene-Environment Interplay: The Questions

Psychiatric disorders cannot be considered in isolation from *behavior.* Genetic factors only explain a fraction of the differences in behavior that may, under some circumstances, result in behavioral disorders. *Psychiatric genetics* is an approach to understanding all the different factors—genetic and environmental, innate and learned, internal and external, physical and social—that explain why some people develop psychiatric disorders and others do not. Studying the effects of genes helps us find out more about the environment and vice versa. Some questions are more obviously "genetic," and some are more typically "environmental." However, humans' capacity to learn and create their world produces a large number of questions that can be answered only by considering both genes and environment at the same time.

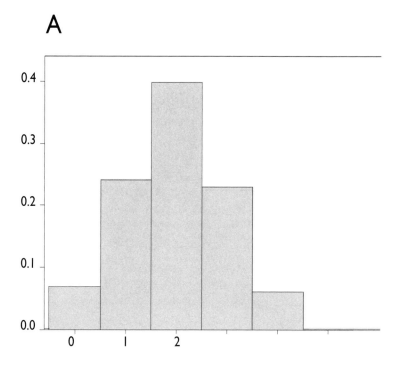

A

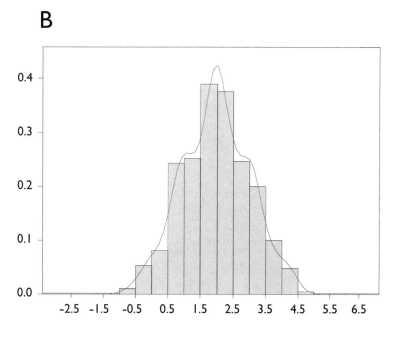

B

C

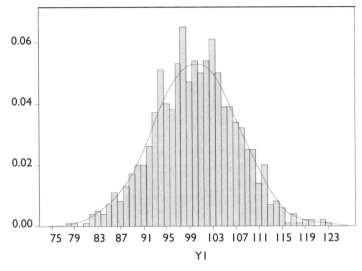

Figure 2–3. Cumulative effects of many genes creating continuous variation.
(A) Distribution of scores produced by two genes (N = 1,000 subjects).
(B) "Smoothing" effect of the environment (N = 1,000 subjects, two-gene model). **(C)** Continuous distribution of polygenic trait (100 genes with small cumulative effects).

"Genetic" Questions

The earliest scientific attempts to understand the role of heredity in human behavior took place more than a century ago with Francis Galton's 1869 study *Hereditary Genius* and Karl Pearson's (1903, 1904) enquiry "On the Laws of Inheritance in Man." At that point, the burning question was, How important are genetic factors in behavioral differences? With this goal still in mind, the 1960s and 1970s were characterized by many studies of large numbers of measures taken from relatively small samples of twins and nuclear families. The 1980s and 1990s saw the explosion of very large studies that used population-based samples to gain much-needed power. It may be that the early 2000s will witness the further transformation of psychiatric genetics by our growing ability to characterize genetic variation and gene expression at incredibly large numbers of genes in very large samples of people. Such developments will require further ingenuity in the design and statistical analysis of psychiatric genetic studies.

Almost every behavioral measure ever devised has, at some time, been administered to a sample of monozygotic (MZ) and dizygotic (DZ) twins in order to provide an estimate of heritability. Criticisms of the "twin method" aside, this groundbreaking work has suggested that the almost all human behavioral traits are affected partly by genetic factors (religious affiliation appears to be a notable exception). The contributions of genetic differences to individual traits may vary as a function of cultural context, the amount of underlying genetic and environmental diversity, and the population's structure, mating system, and history. It usually makes no sense to speak of *the* heritability of a trait.

Some critics (e.g., Feldman and Lewontin 1975) have emphasized the relative crudity of the information derived from these studies and regarded it as shedding little light on the mechanisms underlying the development of human behavior, at the cost of mistakenly reinforcing a number of relatively damaging political and social prejudices. However, this early work laid a critical foundation for a research program that continues to engender significant new insights into the complex interplay between genes and environment in the development of behavior.

The *genetic* aspect of psychiatric genetics is now trying to address a number of more refined questions that go far beyond showing whether behavior is "genetic":

1. How many genes affect particular psychiatric outcomes? Are there a few genes of large effect or large numbers of genes of small effect?
2. If there are genes of large effect, where in the genome are they located and what do they do?
3. How do the effects of multiple genes combine to produce the phenotype? Does each gene just simply add or subtract its own effect to the total (*additive genetic effects*), or do the effects of each gene depend on other genes in the system (*nonadditive genetic effects*)? For example, are there multiple redundant pathways from genes to outcome that buffer the outcome against

adverse changes? Are there chains of cascading genetic effects so that genes later in a pathway are affected by those higher in the chain? Are there several genes or variants within genes that can produce a particular psychiatric disorder (*genetic heterogeneity*)? Do these genes produce exactly the same disorder or somewhat different syndromes?

4. Do genetic effects depend on sex? For example, do different genes affect males and females differently (*sex limitation*)? Do the same genes affect different behavioral traits in males and females? Are any genetic effects on behavior linked to the sex chromosomes (*sex linkage*)? Does the effect of genetic variants on offspring depend on which parent they were inherited from (*imprinting*)? Do genetic differences in mothers, for example, affect the environment of offspring (*maternal effects*)?

5. Do some genetic effects influence multiple outcomes (*comorbidity, genetic covariance, pleiotropy*)? For example, is the correlation between anxiety and depression the result of a common underlying genetic liability? To what extent do genetic effects on antisocial behavior contribute to genetic risk to substance use and abuse?

6. To what extent do different genes affect different outcomes (*trait-specific genetic effects*)?

7. How do the effects of genes unfold over time? Do the same genes affect behavior over long periods of life, or do different genes affect an outcome at different ages? Are the behavioral effects of the same genes different at different developmental stages?

8. To what extent can genetic influences on complex behavioral outcomes be resolved into their effects on simpler, or more elementary, traits at the cellular or neurobiological level (*endophenotypes*)?

9. Can the organization, effects, and functional relationships of genes affecting behavior further elucidate the adaptive role of behavior in human evolution?

"Environmental" Questions

Parallel to the genetic questions is a series of questions concerning environmental influences. Some of these questions are complements of the genetic questions asked above, but many influence specific methods chosen for the design and analysis of particular psychiatric genetic studies.

1. How important are nongenetic effects on particular outcomes?
2. To what extent are the environmental effects shared by family members, and to what extent are they unique to individual offspring within the family?
3. Are "shared" environmental effects created by parents? Are they influenced by other persons or factors (teachers, siblings, peers, exposure to media, etc.)?
4. Do environmental influences have a lasting effect on psychiatric outcomes, or are their effects relatively transient? That is, are people permanently traumatized by experience, or do they recover from adversity?
5. What are the specific environmental influences on particular outcomes? To what extent do these result from social learning, and to what extent do they result from physical experience (accident, infection, pre- and perinatal events)?
6. Are there developmental stages during which some environmental effects are especially salient? Are there sensitive periods in psychological development?
7. Do the effects of environmental factors affect multiple outcomes (*environmental covariance*), or are they specific to particular outcomes? Which particular environments influence which specific outcomes?

Gene-Environment Interplay

Modern psychiatric genetics cannot ignore the environment any more than developmental and social psychology can ignore the genes. Treating genes and environment in isolation from each other may lead us to miss essential characteristics of *human* behavior and its disorders. Humans have a remarkable facility to create and evaluate their environment—a process that primarily involves providing extended parental care and living together in families and other complex social groups. Human development is a conversation between genes and their environment that modifies the expression of genes and shapes the environment in which development occurs. Such reciprocal effects generate relationships between genetic and environmental influences that are referred to frequently as *gene-environment interplay.*

Gene-environment interplay (see, e.g., Rutter and Silberg 2001; Silberg and Rutter 2001) encompasses mechanisms that a social psychologist might refer to under the general heading of *social* interaction and that geneticists would include under the heading of *genotype × environment* interaction. The concept embraces those mechanisms that often depend on the behavior of the whole person and of those who are genetically related to that person. Such effects of the "extended phenotype" (Dawkins 1982) reflect ways in which genetic influences (and hence natural selection) extend beyond the boundaries of the individual into the social and material world.

There are two broad types of gene-environment interplay. First, genetic differences between people may affect the environments they choose or experience (*genotype-environment correlation,* or rGE). Second, genetic differences may change sensitivity to environmental influences (*genotype × environment interaction,* or G×E). In nonhuman organisms, G×E is shown by those genes that affect sensitivity to specific features of the environment, such as temperature, density, and rainfall. By contrast, genotype-environment correlation may arise when the genes of mothers become the environments of offspring. Identification of specific genes or environments and understanding of behavioral development require tools that resolve these processes in which the roles of genes and environment are harder to separate. We discuss the mechanisms of gene-environment interplay in more detail below.

Richard Dawkins (1982) coined the term "extended phenotype" for those human qualities that reflect the extension of genetic effects into the highest reaches of culture and human behavior. The behavior of one person toward another may be influenced by characteristics that are partly genetic, subject to change and fine-tuning by natural selection. The extended phenotype (see Figure 2–4) offers a conceptual framework for thinking about the many ways in which the effects of a person's genes reach beyond their immediate impact on physique and behavior into the world around them.

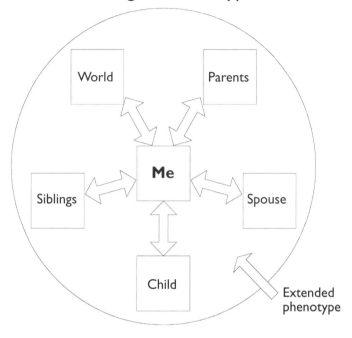

Extending the Phenotype

Figure 2–4. The extended phenotype.

The Place of the "Model" in Psychiatric Genetics

As in most fields of scientific research, psychiatric genetics involves a long-term conversation between question, model, and method (Figure 2–5). A good model puts together what we already know and guides our research in the future. The molecular structure of DNA (the "double helix") is a model that focused almost 100 prior years of biological study, and it has created more than half a century of science since. Models are abstractions that may comprise flowcharts or mathematical equations that summarize one or more ideas about the pathways from genes to behavior.

The models we develop differ from those in pure mathematics or logic because they are designed to lead to the accumulation of critical observations that test our predictions against the real

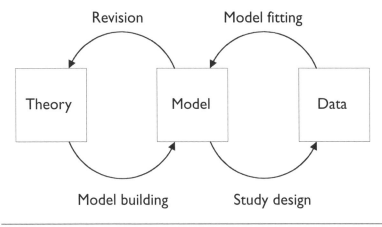

Revision   Model fitting

| Theory | Model | Data |

Model building   Study design

Figure 2–5. The model-fitting approach to psychiatric genetics.

world. Good models have heuristic value. They facilitate development of methods (experiments, measurements, surveys), the results of which encourage us to ask new and more profound questions in an attempt to probe more deeply into the mechanisms underlying human behavior.

Many psychologists have learned to call this approach the *hypothetico-deductive* method and often regard it as the gold standard for inquiry ("true" science). However, much that is challenging in modern genetics stems from *discovery science* analogous to the natural history of old, in which simply describing organisms uncovered unimagined features and patterns of nature that could not have been foreseen if science had been governed simply by the hypothetico-deductive method. Indeed, discovery science rather than the hypothetico-deductive method would seem to have been the root of Charles Darwin's development of the theory of evolution. The power of this theory to make accurate predictions and explain an enormous variety of biological, archaeological, and social phenomena is quite extraordinary.

The task of comparing the results of a study with predictions based on the model is sometimes called *model-fitting* (see, e.g., Eaves et al. 1978). In many classical experiments, effects were either "there" or "not there." In most studies of behavior, however, differences are often small and obscured by the effects of chance and other factors. This means that model-fitting in almost all of psychiatric genetics requires statistical methods that allow us to evaluate the effects, large or small, of chance on experimental findings. We outline some of the basic statistical concepts later in this chapter.

Beyond Words: Modeling Nature and Nurture

If questions are to be answered, ideas have to engage data. Questions must be translated into formal models and into studies that yield the data to test specific hypotheses. The *multifactorial* character of human differences (i.e., the fact that measured differences in behavior reflect large numbers of causal factors) means that we need an approach that embraces the many shades of variation that we encounter in behavior-genetic studies. Inevitably, psychiatric genetics is *quantitative,* and its mode of creative expression is necessarily *mathematical and statistical.* We illustrate in the sections that follow some of the basic ideas that underlie the statistical models of psychiatric genetics; for a more extended treatment, the motivated reader should consult technical texts and articles (e.g., Falconer and Mackay 1996; Ferreira 2004; Jinks and Fulker 1970; Mather and Jinks 1982; Neale and Cardon 1992; Ott 1999; Thomas 2004).

Genes and Environment: Path Models

In the 1920s Sewall Wright (1921) developed *path analysis* as a convenient way of crystallizing ideas about the relationships among multiple variables. Wright's approach has been widely used in behavioral and psychiatric genetics to represent models for the effects of genes and environment on behavioral outcomes. Path analysis is a convenient and flexible *conceptual* tool, because it provides a set of rules for summarizing complex hypotheses in a diagrammatic form—the so-called path diagram. Once a relatively simple set of conventions is adopted, investigators can communicate and criticize their different models for a particular set of outcomes. Beyond that, Wright's approach, combined with the power of modern statistics and computing, provides a mathematical foundation for *testing models* for the patterns of correlation that are expected in real data. Wright's genius was to develop a diagrammatic approach and a set of elementary rules that, used in conjunction with the diagram, would yield correct algebraic expressions for predicted correlations without explicit use of more abstract (and less familiar) mathematical devices. *Path analysis* is an older term for what has become known more generally as "structural equation modeling" (Bollen 1989). Many statistical methods familiar to clinical researchers, such as multiple linear regression, analysis of variance, discriminant function, and factor analysis, turn out to be special cases of the more general approach of structural equation modeling.

Figure 2–6 shows an example of a "genetic" path model that illustrates many features of path diagrams. By convention, variables that are actually measured (such as personality) are shown in squares. Thus, in the diagram, the phenotype is shown in the box labeled *P*. Unmeasured theoretical constructs that explain the variation and relationship among the observed measures— so-called latent variables—are represented by circles. In the example, differences in the measured phenotype, *P*, from the overall mean are shown as "caused by" latent genetic differences, *G*, and environmental influences, *E*. *G* and *E* are latent variables and so are shown in circles. Beyond identifying the measured and latent variables, the path diagram also represents our hypothesis about how the variables are related. The hypothesized direction of causation is represented by single-headed arrows. There is a single-headed arrow from *G* to *P* because we think of genetic differences as causing differences in the phenotype. Similarly, there is a single-headed arrow from *E* to *P*.

Many early genetic models assumed that genes and environment were independent of each other—that is, there was no "genotype-environment" correlation. However, in free-living social organisms, we expect that the effects of the environment will covary with those of the genes for a variety of reasons. In the path diagram, we admit this possibility by including a double-headed arrow between *G* and *E*. The double-headed arrow means that there is a covariance between causes that needs to be considered but that we are not committing ourselves to any specific hypothesis about its cause (that would require extending the diagram further back). Similarly, a double-headed arrow from a variable to itself represents intrinsic variation in that variable—covariation with itself—that is not accounted for by causal paths coming from other variables. These double-headed arrows are typically standardized to unit variance for latent variables.

The third layer of the path model comprises the actual quantities (*path coefficients*) that represent the relative importance of the different causal pathways and the strength of the covariances represented by the double-headed arrows. The quantities h and e alongside the single-headed arrows are the *path coefficients* that represent the relative contributions of differences in G and E to the phenotype. The path coefficients correspond to the partial regression coefficients familiar in multiple regression analysis (though in the usual multiple regression all relevant variables are assumed to be measured directly and there are no "latent" variables).

The strength of the hypothesized genotype-environment covariance is represented by the variable r in the diagram alongside the two-headed arrow between G and E. At the stage of model building, the actual values of path coefficients are unknown and are represented by algebraic constants written alongside the arrows in the path diagram. Ultimately, we want to assign numerical quantities to these relative contributions. This is the statistical task of "estimation" (see below) conducted as part of the model-fitting process.

Structural equation modeling offers enormous conceptual strengths. It provides an elegant way of representing concepts about how genes and environment contribute to human differences and family resemblance. Path analysis remains the most flexible framework for visualizing many complex features that affect human differences. Among other things, models have been developed to represent social interaction with parents (Eaves and Silberg, in press), siblings, (Carey 1986), and children and peers; nongenetic inheritance (Rice et al. 1978); the contribution of measured and latent environmental effects (Neale and Cardon 1992); sex differences in gene expression (Truett et al. 1994); assortative mating (Heath et al. 1985); developmental change (Boomsma and

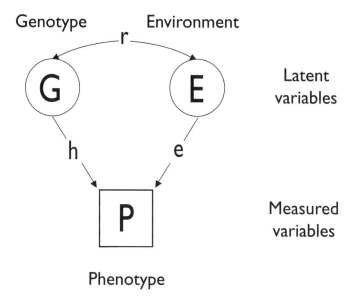

Genotype   Environment

G   r   E

Latent variables

h   e

P

Measured variables

Phenotype

Figure 2–6. Path model for effects of genes and environment on phenotype.
See text for details.

Molenaar 1987; Eaves et al. 1986); the causes of correlation between multiple measures (Neale and Cardon 1992); and genetic linkage and association (Allison and Neale 2002; Neale 2001). However, no one approach can provide all the answers, and we need to be aware of limitations and alternatives.

A common limitation of most (but not all) structural equation models is that they are additive. For example, in Figure 2–6 it is assumed that the phenotype can be approximated by adding together the effects of genes and environment; that is, this particular path model ignores G×E. Although "nonadditive" latent variable models have been devised for some time (Schumaker and Marcoulides 1998), they have not been widely used in practice, and some of them require different computational techniques from those used for exploring additive models. In this basic path model, additivity is represented by the assumption that the path coefficients are constant across people. For example, the sensitivity of individuals to environmental effects, e, is the same for all genotypes. G×E arises when the path *e*, from *E* to *P*, is no longer constant but depends on genotype (or because the path *h*, from *G* to *P*, depends on environment). Similarly, this basic path model construes the effects of individual genetic differences on *G* as cumulative and additive. It assumes that genes and alleles do not interact with each other (i.e., that the effect of one gene does not depend on variation in other genes). However, different forms of the same gene may interact with one another (*dominance*), and the effect of one gene may depend on differences at other genes (*epistasis*). Linear structural models lead to mathematically convenient approaches to statistical analysis. By contrast, the statistical and computational methods required for models that incorporate G×E and gene × gene interactions are more challenging and still in their relative infancy.

Finding the Genes: Quantitative Trait Loci (QTLs)

The historical separation of the multifactorial/polygenic approach to human differences from the approach that tries to break the genetic component down into individual genes of large effect reflects partly a difference in focus and partly a difference in underlying assumptions about the nature of variation in behavior. Linkage and association studies assume that at least some of the individual genetic effects are large enough to stand out against the background of other genetic and environmental variation (quantitative trait loci, or QTLs; see Figure 2–3, panels A and B). Multifactorial/polygenic approaches have focused on the epigenetic rules that govern the integration of genetic and environmental effects at the phenotypic level, and of the developmental and social effects often ignored in other, more molecular, genetic approaches to behavior.

These approaches must be integrated. Identification of individual genetic variants at the molecular level stimulates attempts to find out how these individual genes affect behavior. The growing recognition of the large number of genes affecting the long and complex path from DNA to behavior, and of the role of nongenetic factors at every level, demands approaches that incorporate the effects of many genes and environmental influences into a single model. Structural equation modeling provides a common framework for discussing all kinds of genetic and environmental effects, including those of QTLs on complex traits. Linkage and association studies (see subsection "Finding the Genes: Linkage and Association" later in this chapter) offer two methods for finding individual genes that have different strengths and weaknesses.

From DNA to Behavior: Endophenotypes and Development

The complexity of the path from genes and behavior means that trying to identify genes while ignoring the intermediate stages in the pathway may not work. There are two basic approaches to bridging the gap between DNA and psychopathology. One approach is to study *development* in the hope that earlier behavior will mediate the roles of genes and environment on the trajectory from birth to behavioral outcome. This approach reflects an assumption that later disorder reflects processes that can be dissected into components that are ordered sequentially in time. Developmental studies in psychiatric genetics follow the behavior and environment of genetically informative samples (e.g., twins or high-risk children). The longitudinal developmental approach may help tease apart the unfolding developmental feedback between genetic and environmental influences (person-environment interplay). A second approach is to study other variables and processes that may intervene between the cellular and behavioral level, known as *endophenotypes.* These measures "within" the organism are thought to mediate the effects of genes on complex outcomes at a more fundamental level (see, e.g., Hasler et al. 2004). Endophenotypes may include levels of gene expression; biological markers such as indicators of metabolic function; hypothesized intervening behavioral variables such as personality; or neurobiological assessments of brain structure and function. The methods of *multivariate genetic analysis* (see subsection "Multiple Variables" later in this chapter) provide a framework for modeling the relationships between endophenotypes and psychopathology.

The endophenotype concept is illustrated by the path diagram in Figure 2–7. Variation in risk to the outcome depends partly on measured endophenotypes (P_1–P_4) and partly on residual unmeasured, latent effects of genes and environment. Similarly,

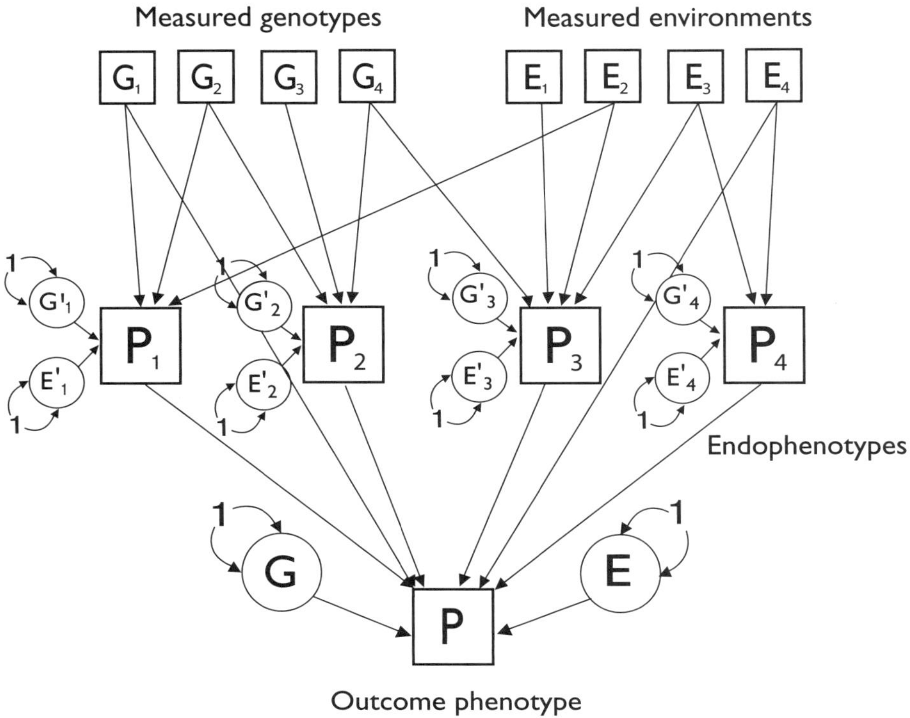

Figure 2–7. Illustrative model for the role of endophenotypes in mediating the effects of genes and environments on complex outcomes.

each endophenotype reflects the effects of genes and environment. Some of the genetic and environmental effects are measured explicitly (G_1–G_4, E_1–E_4), and some are unmeasured latent variables (e.g., G'_1, E'_4). In addition, there may be relationships among the endophenotypes that reflect cascades of intervening variables. To the extent that psychiatric genetics seeks to identify and measure the specific genetic and environmental processes that contribute to risk, endophenotypes may be helpful if they are closer to the function of fewer specific genes than the complex outcome. Whether this is the case remains to be established.

Family Resemblance and the Correlations Between Relatives

Measures of variation by themselves cannot distinguish between the effects of genes and those of the environment. Methods are needed that allow us to estimate the effects of both. Francis Galton (1883) realized, in his *Inquiry Into Human Faculty and Its Development,* that twins provided the lever he needed, and Ronald Fisher in 1918 provided some of the statistical framework needed in his paper on the correlation between relatives. Key to this early development was the *correlation coefficient,* a statistic originally devised by Galton to provide a measure of association between continuous measures and applied by Pearson, Lee, and others in the first decade of the twentieth century to measure *the correlations between relatives* (Pearson and Lee 1903). The correlation quantifies the degree of association between pairs of measures that can be visualized graphically in a scatter diagram. Different study designs offer opportunities to focus more strongly on one or the other feature of diathesis and stress. Some are more powerful for genetic analysis, whereas others offer greater power for exploring the environment and the extended phenotype. Whatever the design, however, a common conceptual thread is the modeling and analysis of *patterns of family resemblance* reflected in the correlations between relatives.

Figure 2–8 shows scatter diagrams for stature in DZ and MZ pairs, respectively, after stature is expressed as a deviation from the main for the corresponding age and sex. The diagrams show the patterns of association between relatives showing high (MZ

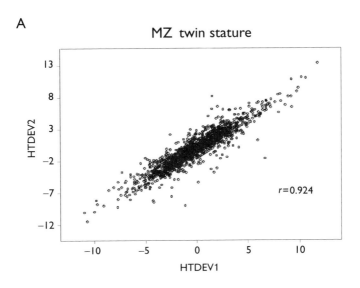

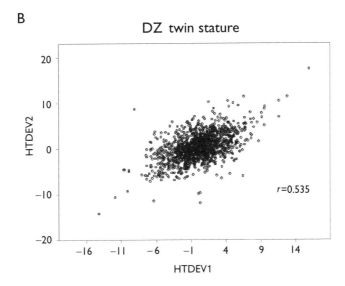

Figure 2–8. Correlation between twins for stature.

(A) Scatterplot for age- and sex-corrected stature in MZ twins. **(B)** Scatterplot for age- and sex-corrected stature in DZ twins.

Note. Stature expressed as deviation from corrected means for first (HTDEV1) and second (HTDEV2) twins.

Source. Data from the Virginia Twin Study of Adolescent Behavioral Development.

twins: $r = 0.924$) and intermediate (DZ twins: $r = 0.535$) correlation. A correlation of zero would show a circular scatter of points. Fisher (1918) and a series of researchers since then (e.g., Fulker 1988; Heath et al. 1985; Jencks 1972; Jinks and Fulker 1970; Morton 1974; Neale and Cardon 1992; Rice et al. 1978; Truett et al. 1994) have provided a variety of different models for the effects of genes and environment on family resemblance. Many of these models have been motivated by a need to account for the unique patterns of family resemblance to be expected in behavioral traits and disorders.

Resolving the Effects of Genes and Environment: Twin Studies

In typical nuclear family studies, the effects of genetic inheritance are inextricably entwined with the effects of the environment passed between family members. Long before it was possible to type people for genetic markers, Galton realized that identical twins are produced by the division into two of a single zygote after fertilization. Galton recognized that for most practical purposes, such *monozygotic twins* were "genetically" identical (the word *gene* was unknown for another 50 years) but had different environmental experiences. He appreciated the value of twins as a natural experiment. Differences between the life histories and behavior of identical twins were an indicator of the relative importance of nongenetic effects. Non-identical twins (or fraternal twins) arose because two separate eggs were released from their mother's ovary at the same time and fertilized by two different sperm. Thus, although such *dizygotic twins* shared part of their genetic material in common because they had the same parents, they were not identical because, like brothers and sisters, each carried a unique sample of their parental genes. Dizygotic twins, therefore, were genetically correlated but not genetically identical and provided a control for the natural experiment of monozygotic twins.

The extent to which identical twins are different is a measure of the effects of the environment unique to each twin (now referred to as the *unique* environment, *E,* or the *within-family* environment), because it reflects those environmental differences

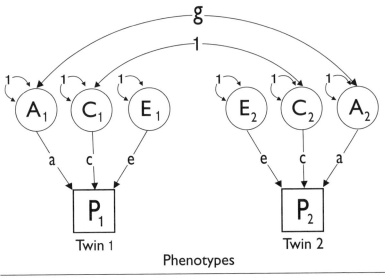

Figure 2–9. One path model for twin resemblance.
See text for details.

within the family that make one family member differ from another. To the extent that dizygotic twins are less alike than monozygotic twins, the natural conclusion is that genetic factors are important. One measure of their importance is the difference between the two correlations.

Path Model for Twin Resemblance

The path model for the effects of genes and environment on phenotypic differences may be extended to the causes of resemblance between twins (Figure 2–9).

The model has two manifest variables, the *trait values of first and second twins*, P_1 and P_2, respectively, and three latent variables that may influence the phenotype of each twin. The effects of the environment are divided into those that are correlated between twins—the "common," "shared," or "between-family" environments of first and second twins, C_1 and C_2, respectively—and those that are uncorrelated across twin pairs—the unique, "specific," "individual," or "within-family" environments, E_1 and $E_2.$ The initial model for the latent genetic effects assumes that the effects of alleles and loci are additive (i.e., there are no nonadditive genetic effects). A common convention denotes the latent additive genetic effects of the two twins by A_1 and A_2, respectively. This model, commonly referred to as the *ACE model*, constitutes a convenient starting point for the discussion of twin and family resemblance (see, e.g., Neale and Cardon 1992).

Although the within-family environmental effects in Figure 2–9, E_1 and E_2, are assumed to be uncorrelated, the same is not true for the genetic effects, A_1 and A_2, or for the shared family environments, C_1 and C_2. The C components reflect all pre- and postnatal influences that twins share by virtue of developing in the same family. We thus assume that C_1 and C_2 are completely and equally correlated between twins regardless of zygosity. The correlation between shared environmental effects is shown in the diagram by the double-headed arrow between C_1 and C_2. This arrow implies that, although C_1 and C_2 are correlated, neither causes the other. The correlation coefficient alongside the double-headed arrow is set to 1 *ex hypothesi*. The correlation between genetic effects is expected to be different in MZ and DZ twins. In the diagram, we denote this correlation by g. Since MZ twins are genetically identical, $g = 1$ in MZ twins. In DZ twins, g will be less than 1 depending on the mating system and exactly how the genes operate. If there is no assortative mating and if the effects of genes are purely additive, $g = \frac{1}{2}$ in DZ twins.

The path diagram is a graphical version of a structural equation model (Bollen 1989; see subsection "Genes and Environment: Path Models" earlier in this section). Wright developed a set of convenient *tracing rules* that translate the task of deriving algebraic formulas for variances and correlations into fairly simple procedures that yield the correct answers without the need for more abstract matrix algebra. In the simplest case, such as that in Figure 2–9, we assume that the manifest and latent variables are all standardized to unit variance. Since the actual units of measurement are often arbitrary and of little interest, standardization does not usually sacrifice any important properties of the data in this simple case.

If the variables are all standardized, then the formula for the expected correlation between P_1 and P_2 is given by the following set of rules:

1. Start from one of the two variables of interest (e.g., P_1).
2. Trace every possible pathway from P_1 to P_2 subject to the following restrictions: a) trace backward any number (zero or more) of steps, change direction at a double-headed arrow, and then go forward any number (zero or more) of steps; b) never go backward again having ever gone forward; and c) change direction only once.
3. Accumulate the contributions of all possible pathways (see below) to generate the formula for the desired correlation.

In Figure 2–9 there are two distinct pathways from P_1 to P_2: $P_1 \rightarrow A_1 \rightarrow A_2 \rightarrow P_2$ and $P_1 \rightarrow C_1 \rightarrow C_2 \rightarrow P_2$. The contribution of each pathway to the twin correlation is the product of the coefficients beside all the arrows in that pathway. Thus, the first path contributes $a \times g \times a = ga^2$, and the second path contributes $c \times 1 \times c = c^2$. The final formula for the twin correlation is simply the sum of these contributions:

$$r_{twin} = ga^2 + c^2$$

The first part of the correlation, ga^2, is the contribution of additive polygenic factors. The second part, c^2, is the contribution of the shared environment. The unique environment, E, makes no contribution to the correlation because the independence of E_1 and E_2 means that there is no path (i.e., no double-headed arrow) between them.

Substituting the appropriate value for g in the above general formula gives the expression for the correlation of each type of twins:

for MZ pairs,

$$r_{MZ} = a^2 + c^2$$

and for DZ pairs,

$$r_{DZ} = \tfrac{1}{2}a^2 + c^2$$

The third equation implied by the model is that for the total phenotypic variance, V_P. Since the total variance is standardized to unity, the expectation is given by the following formula:

$$V_P = 1 = a^2 + c^2 + e^2$$

The model described above makes several assumptions: 1) additive gene action; 2) random mating; 3) no G×E interaction; 4) no genotype-environment correlation; 5) autosomal inheritance; 6) environmental effects comparable and equally correlated in MZ and DZ twins (the *equal environments assumption*, or EEA); 7) no mutual influence of twins (i.e., no competition, contrast, mutual reinforcement, or cooperation between the phenotypes of twins; Eaves 1976); and 8) same genetic and environmental effects across sexes and ages.

The sample of twins is assumed to be representative of the population of genetic and environmental effects. If the sample is not random but selected on the basis of the phenotype of one or both twins or on some correlated variable, the above expectations will not apply and the analysis must be adjusted accordingly. Assumptions are designed to be tested. The task of model-building is to make such assumptions explicit and to provide a framework of analysis so that they may be tested where possible.

The foregoing equations for the correlations of MZ and DZ twins predict different patterns of twin correlation under different models for the contributions of genes and environment to individual differences. Figure 2–10 illustrates four of the simple possibilities. In the diagram, the heights of the bars represent possible correlations for MZ and DZ twins.

In the first case (No *A*), the bars for MZ and DZ twins are the same height—a scenario that we would expect to find if there were no genetic effects on the trait but large effects of the shared environment (*C*). The fact that the MZ correlation is less than 1 tells us that there are effects of the within-family environment (*E*) that make even identical twins differ even though they share the same genes, the same mother, and the same overall home environment. The second scenario shows what we would expect to find if there were additive genetic effects (*A*) but no effects of the shared environment (No *C*). The DZ correlation is much less than the MZ correlation and, when the genetic effects are additive, equal to half the MZ correlation. In practice, the effects of chance cause, in specific cases, correlations to vary from what is expected. Statistical-genetic analysis helps us decide when the differences between observed and predicted patterns are most likely a mat-

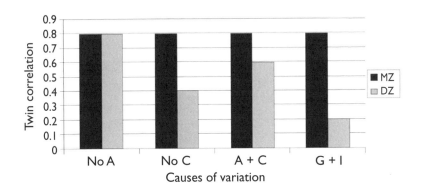

Figure 2–10. Patterns of twin correlations under four models for genetic and environmental effects.

DZ = dizygotic twin; MZ = monozygotic twin.

ter of chance fluctuations and when they are due to real effects that need to be included in a model. The third scenario in the figure depicts what we would expect to find if both genes and shared environment caused family resemblance (*A* and *C*). Now the MZ correlation is greater than the DZ correlation, but the DZ correlation exceeds half the MZ correlation. The fourth scenario depicts the pattern of twin correlations we would expect to find if there were large nonadditive genetic effects due to epistasis or dominance (I). In every case, the precise pattern of correlations to be expected depends on the exact contributions of the various genetic and environmental factors and, in the case of genetic effects, on the exact pattern of allele frequencies, and on the magnitudes of the specific additive, dominance, and epistatic effects at individual genes and gene combinations.

First Estimates of Genetic and Environmental Effects on Stature

Figure 2–8 presents the scatter diagrams and correlations for stature in MZ and DZ twins. The MZ correlation (0.924) is close to 1, and the DZ correlation (0.535) is quite close to half the MZ correlation. Comparing the correlations with the correlation patterns in Figure 2–10 suggests that the raw correlations look very much like those in the second scenario (No C).

Writing our three equations again and inserting the observed twin correlations, we have

$$r_{MZ} = a^2 + c^2 = 0.924 \quad (1)$$

$$r_{DZ} = \tfrac{1}{2}a^2 + c^2 = 0.535 \quad (2)$$

and

$$V_P = 1 = a^2 + c^2 + e^2 \quad (3)$$

The three equations yield estimates of the contributions of a^2, c^2, and e^2 to the total variation in stature: $\hat{a}^2 = 0.778$, $c^2 = 0.146$, and $\hat{e}^2 = 0.076$. The caret symbol (^) is used to denote the estimate of a parameter derived from data. Thus, initial estimates for this age group suggest that, after removal of the effects of age and sex, almost 78% of the variation in stature is due to the additive effects of genes, approximately 8% is due to within-family environmental effects, and the remaining 14%–15% is due to effects of the shared family environment. Although the current data do not allow us to explore the effects of assortative mating, some of what we have estimated as c^2 in this simple analysis could be due to the *genetic* consequences of the modest assortative mating observed for stature.

Adoption Studies: Another Approach to Separating Genes and Environment

Adoption usually refers to the rearing of a child in a family whose members are not related to the child biologically. This practice is commonplace after wars, which leave many children orphaned, and is moderately frequent in peacetime. Approximately 2% of U.S. citizens are adoptees. Historically, adoption studies have played a prominent role in the assessment of genetic variation in human and animal traits. Adopting families in which at least one member is not biologically related to the others offer a number of potential comparisons that can be genetically informative. Thus, the correlation of adoptees with their biological parents is a reflection of the *genetic* contribution of parents to their children. The correlation between children and their adopting (biologically unrelated) parents reflects the environmental effects of parents on children.

Adoption studies may include both biological and adopted children of the foster parents, permitting a direct assessment of the effect of the home environment on the similarity of unrelated children reared together. Heath et al. (1985) compared the power to detect genetic and environmental transmission across several twin–family (twins and their parents or twins and their children) and adoption designs. The conceptual power of the adoption study is enhanced greatly when the study is integrated in a longitudinal multivariate design and includes rich assessments of biological and foster parents as well as of the environment in the foster home.

Most (e.g., Plomin and DeFries 1985) but not all (Heston 1966) of the early adoption studies focused on cognitive abilities, but since then there has been greater emphasis on psychopathology (Cadoret 1978; Cadoret et al. 1986; Cloninger et al. 1981) and physical characteristics such as body mass (Sorensen 1995). Adoption studies have made major substantial contributions to these areas, allowing researchers to identify the effects of genetic factors that were previously thought to be absent. In recent years the adoption study has been overshadowed by the much more popular twin study. Part of this shift may be due to the convenience of twin studies and the complex ethical and legal issues involved in the ascertainment and sampling of adoptees. Certain Scandinavian countries, especially Denmark, Sweden, and Finland (Kaprio et al. 1984; Kety 1987; Pedersen et al. 1991), maintain centralized databases of adoptions, and thus researchers have been able to mount more representative and larger adoption studies in these regions than elsewhere.

The adoption study is a "natural experiment" that mirrors cross-fostering designs used in genetic studies of animals (Mather and Jinks 1982) and that, therefore, has a high face validity as a method of resolving the effects of genes and environment on individual differences. Unfortunately, the adoption study also has many methodological difficulties.

1. *Need to maintain confidentiality.* Diffculties in maintaining confidentiality can arise even at initial ascertainment, as some adoptees do not know they were adopted.
2. *Sampling.* In adoption studies, the potential for sampling bias has an impact in many substantive areas (e.g., psychopathology). Neither the biological parents nor the adoptive parents can be assumed to be a random sample of parents in the population. For example, poverty and its sequelae may be more common among biological parents who have their children adopted into other families than among parents who rear their children themselves. Conversely, prospective adoptive parents are, on average and through self-selection, older and less fertile than biological parents. In addition, they are often carefully screened by adoption agencies and may be of higher socioeconomic status than nonadoptive parents. Statistical methods (see below) may be used to control for these sampling biases if a random sample of parents is available for comparison.
3. *Selective placement.* The ideal adoption study would, for statistical purposes, have randomly selected adoptees placed at random into randomly selected families in the population. However, there is often a partial matching of the characteristics of the adoptee (e.g., hair and eye color, religion and ethnicity) to those of the adopting family. This common practice, known as *selective placement,* may improve the chances of successful adoption. Statistically, it is necessary to control for the matching as far as possible. Ideally, the matching characteristics used should be recorded and modeled. Usually, such detailed information is not available, so matching is assumed to be based on the variables being studied and is modeled accordingly. These methods are widely used in modern adoption studies (Plomin and DeFries 1985).

The rules of path analysis can be used to derive predicted covariances among the relatives in adoption studies just as they can in other kinds of family data. These expectations may in turn be used in a structural equation modeling program such as Mx (Neale and Cardon 1992; see below) to estimate the parameters using maximum likelihood or some other goodness-of-fit function. Often, simpler models than the one shown will be adequate to account for a particular set of data.

Sex Differences in Genetic Effects

Many disorders show sex differences in prevalence and patterns of family resemblance. After puberty, depression is more prevalent in girls, and antisocial behavior is more prevalent in boys. Continuous traits often also show sex differences in mean, variance, and correlation between relatives. Sex differences in mean or prevalence may be due to genetic and/or environmental effects; it is difficult, if not impossible, to decide between genetic and environmental explanations. However, this is not the case for patterns of family resemblance. In the absence of any sex differences in the expression of genes and environments, the correlations between relatives will be the same regardless of the sexes of the relatives involved. However, there are, in principle, several different ways in which sex can affect the expression of genes: sex linkage, sex limitation, imprinting, and maternal effects. Here, we address only sex-limited gene expression, since it seems to be the most widespread mechanism in studies of human behavior and psychiatric disorders.

Sex-limited gene expression occurs when the phenotypic effect of autosomal genes depends on sex. It is a form of genotype x sex interaction. Sometimes, sex simply magnifies or diminishes the effects of all the genes on a particular trait, leading to sex differences in the amount of genetic variation without any marked effect on the overall correlation between relatives. Often, sex may actually *cause* different genes to be expressed in one or the other sex. The latter may not only produce sex differences in variance but, more importantly, reduce the correlations between unlike-sex relatives compared with like-sex pairs. For example, unlike-sex dizygotic twins or siblings will be less alike than like-sex pairs in the presence of this type of sex-limited gene expression.

Finding the Genes: Linkage and Association

It is one thing to show that genes affect behavior and its disorders, but quite another to identify the specific genes that are involved. Early studies of complex traits in experimental organisms, such as fruit flies, indicated that the genes involved are many in number and widely scattered throughout the genome. We usually have little idea about which specific genes affect an outcome or where they are physically located in the genome. Twenty years ago, the number of genes that had been located on particular human chromosomes was very small and represented only a few genes, such as those for blood groups. The situation has changed radically. The study of genetic variation at the DNA level can now be focused even on the individual "letters" of the genetic code (single-nucleotide polymorphisms, or SNPs). This capability opens up new hope that the hitherto unknown genes affecting pathways to human behavior may one day be identified through their association with other genes of known function and genomic location. Another chapter in this book describes the application of some of these approaches to the study of schizophrenia (see Chapter 3, "Genetics of Schizophrenia"). Here, we outline some of the conceptual issues and place them within the broader context of models and methods for analyzing complex behavioral traits and disorders.

Currently, there are two basic approaches to gene finding. *Linkage studies* are conducted to try to explain some of the genetic correlation between relatives by measuring the correlation between relatives in pairs of individuals grouped according to their correlation for specific genes at known places on the genome (see, e.g., Ferreira 2004). *Association studies* are conducted to try to explain part of genetic risk by testing whether variants at a particular gene are correlated directly with a specific outcome measure (see, e.g., Sham 1997; Thomas 2004). Current genetic and statistical technology allows us to scan large numbers of genes to pick out those that seem to be near genes that affect the outcome of interest (see, e.g., Kruglyak and Lander 1995).

Linkage Studies

Linkage studies may use large multigenerational pedigrees or large numbers of small pedigrees (e.g., sib pairs). Pedigrees may be identified through affected individuals obtained through medical referral or through screening of the wider population. Population-based samples may be prescreened to exclude pedigrees in which affected individuals do not occur or to enrich a sample for families at higher risk. The choice of few large pedigrees or a large number of small pedigrees is dictated in part by how the phenotype is measured and how genes are presumed to influence the phenotype of interest.

Whatever strategy is adopted, the linkage study requires that polymorphic genetic *markers* be selected to "tag" the genome at a wide series of locations. A linkage study of the whole genome may involve, initially, several hundred such markers, and then, depending on results of the initial screen, certain locations may be chosen for more detailed analysis using further markers. Markers in linkage studies are typically chosen for their location and informativeness rather than for any possible functional relationship to the outcome, though this rule is by no means invariably followed if there are good reasons to explore particular genes of known function.

The seminal report on the use of linkage to locate genes affecting complex traits (Haseman and Elston 1972) was published before the ready availability of markers having known locations on the human genome. Similarity between relatives for a marker (or a set of markers close to each other) is used to classify pairs of relatives according to the amount of genetic material they share in the region of the markers. For example, ideal markers allow sibling pairs to be divided into three groups depending on whether they inherited copies of the same allele from both, one, or neither parent. Such pairs are said to share two, one, or zero alleles *identical by descent* (IBD). Pairs that share both alleles IBD are expected to be genetically identical at that specific location. So, at that location, such pairs are like monozygotic twins. Similarly, pairs that share no alleles IBD are like unrelated individuals at that marker location. Other genes, not at the marked location, will contribute the same amount to sibling resemblance regardless of IBD status at the marker.

The essence of linkage analysis then consists of plotting the correlation between relatives as a function of the number or genes IBD for each marker location. Usually, IBD is represented as a proportion, Π, of alleles IBD. Π takes values 0, ½ , and 1 in pairs sharing 0, 1, and 2 alleles IBD, respectively. Figure 2–11

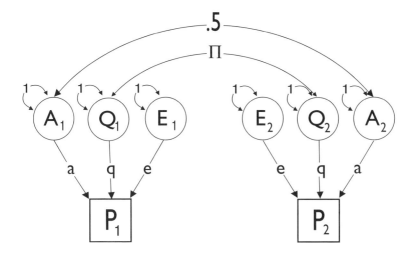

Figure 2–11. Contribution of a quantitative trait locus to sibling resemblance.

The diagram represents a path model for the genetic contribution to sibling pair resemblance with a proportion of alleles IBD, Π. The latent variables, G_1 and G_2, denote the effects of all genes apart from the QTL. Q_1 and Q_2 are the effects of the QTL at the locus of interest. The correlation between the effects of the QTL is Π.

shows a path model for the genetic contribution to sibling pair resemblance with a proportion of alleles IBD, Π. The latent variables, A_1 and A_2, as before, denote the effects of all genes apart from the QTL. Q_1 and Q_2 are the effects of the QTL at the locus of interest. The correlation between the effects of the QTL is Π.

The increase in sibling correlation, r, with increasing IBD, Π, provides a test of linkage between the marker and genes affecting the outcome phenotype (see Figure 2–12). The steeper the increase in r with increasing Π, the larger the effect of the QTL at that location. A *genome scan* tests for the relationship between phenotypic resemblance and Π for markers spread throughout the genome, identifying those locations where there is a significant relationship between r and Π as possible sites for genes affecting the outcome.

In practice, individual markers may not have sufficient variation to provide perfect assignment of every pair to the three IBD

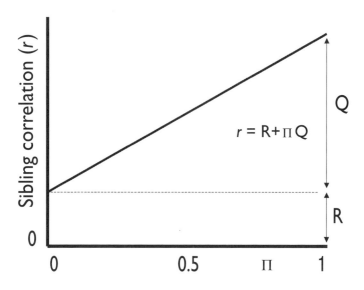

Figure 2–12. Increase in sibling correlation as a function of increased proportion of alleles identical by descent.

classes. Furthermore, r and Π will be less closely associated as the distance between the QTL and the marker increases. *Multipoint mapping* uses the information from large numbers of partly informative markers to increase the precision with which IBD status is assigned and to clarify the location of specific QTLs by exploring the increase or decrease in the relationship between r and Π as the focus moves from one location to the next (Kruglyak and Lander 1995). The approach of correlating r with Π is appropriate in large, population-based studies in which the individuals genotyped are not selected for any particular phenotype. Such a strategy is not cost-effective for relatively rare disorders, such as schizophrenia, or extreme phenotypes. In these cases, kinships are selected on the basis of affected or extreme individuals or combinations of affected individuals. The *affected sib pair* (ASP) method is an example of the use of selected samples—in this case, pairs of siblings selected because both are affected by the disorder. In studies of selected samples, statistical analysis uses the fact that siblings who are alike phenotypically are expected, on average, to be more alike genetically at locations close to QTLs. Similarly, sib pairs who are extremely dissimilar phenotypically are expected to show greater differences genetically at locations nearer QTLs. The selection of kinships on the basis of their phenotype typically recovers much of the information that would be gained from much larger, unselected samples (Risch and Zhang 1995).

Marker Association Studies

Whereas linkage studies explore the correlation between relatives as a function of identity by descent assessed by genetic markers, *association studies* test for a relationship between outcomes and individual alleles at marker loci. Association can be studied in its own right, or jointly with linkage, and may involve genes that are hypothesized to affect the processes that lead to psychopathology ("candidate genes"), such as genes known to affect the activity of neurotransmitters or markers that are used to tag specific locations on the genome. Recently, the concept of *genomewide association*—in which large numbers of markers distributed throughout the genome are examined for possible association with risk to a disorder—has become conceivable. Association studies work if alleles at the marker actually affect susceptibility, or if susceptibility alleles at genes very near the marker are themselves associated nonrandomly with the marker (*linkage disequilibrium*). The advantage of association studies is that under some circumstances, they can detect genes of smaller effects than those detectable in linkage studies. A disadvantage is that the markers have to be much closer to the susceptibility loci for significant association to occur.

The simplest association study is a *case-control study*, in which the frequencies of alleles at marker loci are compared between patients and control subjects. The caveat "correlation does not mean causation" applies as much in genetic association studies as it does in any other epidemiological study. Associations may arise in populations, even between genes on different chromosomes, because of *population stratification*. In the simplest case, a new population produced by aggregating populations with different allele frequencies may show associations between alleles at widely separated genes, even genes on separate chromosomes. Over succeeding generations, with recombination and assortment of genes, the level of association will decline. The effects of recombination cause associations to decay more rapidly for genes that are widely separated in populations in which there is the greatest opportunity for social mobility in mate selection.

The possibility of spurious association leads to a number of strategies for sorting out informative associations due to causal effects of marker alleles or close linkage disequilibrium from those due to population stratification. One set of methods focuses on the fact that associations arising *within families* are free of the effects of stratification. Thus, allele frequencies may be controlled for associations present in the parents—a process known as a *transmission disequilibrium test,* or TDT (Ewens and Spielman 1995; Fulker et al. 1999)—or compared for affected and unaffected siblings within families. Other methods rely on using sets of unrelated markers to estimate and control for the level of association between markers widely separated on the genome as indices of the genetic effects of population stratification.

Finding Genes: Sequence Variation and Genetic Markers

Whether our goal is to locate genes through linkage or association studies, a necessary step is the recognition of genetic differences at the molecular level so these can be correlated, either through linkage or through association, with differences at the phenotypic level. DNA has a double-helix structure and consists of four nucleotides. The combination and order of these four nucleotides code for the functions of genes and other regulatory elements. For humans, our genome has about 3 billion pairs of these nucleotides. While the sequences between individuals are identical for more than 99% of the 3 billion pairs, the less than 1% difference is what makes each of us unique individuals. The sequence variations among individuals are called *polymorphisms* ("many shapes"), and a particular variant is referred to as an *allele.* At any particular location on the genome (known as a *locus*), a person may share zero, one, or two alleles with another person. As the number of polymorphisms or loci increases, the combination of the alleles found in a person becomes less likely to be shared with another person. DNA polymorphisms provide a way to identify and trace a segment of DNA among individuals. This allows researchers to associate a segment of DNA with a specific combination of alleles (also called *haplotype*) to a particular trait. The segment of DNA being studied could be a gene or genes or other elements that predispose or contribute to a disease or a behavior trait. The association of a specific allele or haplotype to a trait provides the basic rationale for linkage and association studies.

There are many different kinds of polymorphisms in DNA. One useful way to classify them is as *insertions, deletions,* and *substitutions.* In each of these cases, the polymorphism may vary greatly in size, from a single base to millions of bases. Large-scale changes, also called *chromosomal rearrangements,* are relatively rare, compared with those that involve only one or tens of bases, and are therefore less useful as genetic markers. The two kinds of polymorphisms commonly used in genetic studies are *variable number tandem repeats* (VNTRs) (also known as *microsatellites*), and *single-nucleotide polymorphisms* (SNPs). VNTR markers, as implied by their name, contain multiple tandem repeats of two, three, four, or five nucleotides. The most commonly seen two-nucleotide repeats (known as *dinucleotides*) are CA repeats. One example, D5S678, is shown in Figure 2–13A, where a string of CA dinucleotides is found between nonrepeating sequences. Many VNTR markers have been mapped in the human genome; a comprehensive list is available from the National Center for Biotechnology Information (NCBI) databases (http://www.ncbi.nlm. nih. gov/genome/guide/human/). For VNTR markers, the number of tandem units repeated defines the alleles. SNPs, on the other hand, are single-nucleotide substitutions at a particular position of a DNA sequence. Because DNA sequences consist of only four nucleotides, the maximal number of alleles is four, and most of them consist of only two alleles.

Figure 2–13B shows an example of a SNP, rs4680, which is in the catechol-*O*-methyltransferase gene located on chromosome 22.

A. D5S678

```
gccccacctg  cccccttatc  cgcccccTac  ccgcccccTt  atccaccccc  50
tacctgcccc  ctcctccatc  tttcattcac  caccctgctt  tgattagtgc  100
agcttcatca  ggagcctagg  agccgggcag  CATGAGTCCC  GTGACTTTGT  150
tcttcaattt  tgtgttggtt  gtgctgggtc  tttcctctct  ctatgtaaac  200
ttcagaatca  tttctcaata  gccacaaaat  aacttgctag  gattttgatt  250
gagtataCAC  ACACACACAC  ACACACACGC  GCGCACACAC  ACACACACAt  300
atttgagatg  ctcctggagt  gcagtgatgc  gatctcggct  tactgcaacc  350
tccacctccc  ggatTCATGC  AATTCTCCTG  CCtcagcctc  gctagtagct  400
ggggttacag  gcgtgtgcca  ccaggcctgg  ctaatttttg  tatttttagt  450
agagatacgg  tttcacaatg  ttggccaggc  tggtctcaat  ctgctgacct  500
```

B. rs4680

```
ggccgtgcct  ggggatccaa  gttcccctct  ctccacctgt  gctcacctct  50
cctccgtccc  caaccctgca  caggcaagat  cgtggacgcc  gtgattcagg  100
agcaccagcc  ctccgtgctG  CTGGAGCTGG  GGGCCTACTg  tggctactca  150
gctgtgcgca  tggcccgcct  gctgtcacca  ggggcgaggc  tcatcaccat  200
cgagatcaac  cccgactgtg  ccgccatcac  ccagcggatg  gtggatttcg  250
ctggc
R
tgaaggacaa  ggtgtgcatg  cctgacccgt  tgtcagacct  ggaaaaaggg  306
ccggctgtgg  gcagggaggg  catgcgcact  ttgtcctccc  caccaggtGT  356
TCACACCACG  TTCACTGAAA  ACCcactatc  accaggcccc  tcagtgcttc  406
ccagcctggg  gctgaggaaa  gacccccca  gcagctcagt  gagggtctca  456
cagctctggg  taaactgcca  aggtggcacc  aggaggggca  gggacagagt  506
ggggc
```

Figure 2–13. Examples of polymorphisms commonly used for genetic studies.

(A) A *variable number tandem repeat* (VNTR) marker, also referred to as a *microsatellite marker,* is a polymorphism that consists of tandem repeats of two, three, four, or more nucleotides. The example shown, D5S678, which contains multiple repeats of CA dinucleotides (bolded italic), is in the 5′ promoter region of the dopamine transporter gene (*DAT1*; also known as *SLC6A3*) located on chromosome 5. The difference in repeating units represents different alleles. (B) In a *single-nucleotide polymorphism* (SNP), more than one nucleotide is observed at a particular position of a DNA sequence. rs4680 is a functional polymorphism in the catechol-*O*-methyltransferase (COMT) gene that involves the adenosine and guanine nucleotide. (R is the standard code for the A/G polymorphism.) Most SNPs are bi-allelic. A pair of polymerase chain reaction primers (underlined and struck through) flanking the polymorphisms is necessary to amplify and genotype both VNTR and SNP markers.

SNP rs4680 has two alleles, A and G, and the change of the nucleotide from A to G, when translated, results in an amino acid change from methionine to valine. This functional change has been implicated in psychiatric disorders such as schizophrenia and bipolar disorder. In the last few years, millions of SNPs have been discovered and have been made available in the NCBI SNP database (http://www.ncbi.nlm.nih.gov/SNP/index.html). Note that the overwhelming majority of SNPs do not result in amino acid changes. Functional SNPs, such as rs4680, account for about 1%–2% of all SNPs discovered.

Microsatellite markers are commonly used for genomewide linkage studies (Weber and Broman 2001). Several marker sets that cover the human genome evenly at 5–30 cM are commercially available. SNPs, on the other hand, are popular for association studies. Several characteristics of SNPs make them suitable for association studies (Cardon and Abecasis 2003; Shastry 2003). First, they are highly frequent in the human genome. Currently, the major SNP database contains more than 5 million SNPs in the human genome, which means that, on average, more than one SNP has been identified for every 1,000 DNA base pairs. Although the distribution of SNPs is not even across the genome, the majority of the human genome is covered with a high density of SNPs. The second valuable feature of SNPs is that they are more stable over evolutionary time (less likely to change) than are VNTR markers. This makes them more suitable for association studies. One weakness of SNPs is that they are less informative, per marker, than VNTRs, because they have only two alleles at a locus. This weakness can be compensated for by using more SNPs.

Molecular Techniques for Genotyping

Polymerase chain reaction. The invention of the polymerase chain reaction (PCR), a technique for amplifying a DNA segment in vitro, caused a revolution in molecular biology. PCR uses heat to separate the two strands of the DNA double helix and then employs a pair of short oligonucleotides, known as *primers,* to synthesize two new strands, using the two old strands as templates. In this process, the amount of targeted DNA fragment doubles for each cycle. The discovery of thermally stable DNA polymerases made this process robust and practical. When the process is repeated 30–40 times, the amount of targeted DNA increases by a factor of over a million. Because a genetic marker occupies a unique position in the genome, it accounts for only a tiny fraction of total genomic DNA. For this reason, amplification of targeted regions of the genome has become an essential part of genotyping protocols.

Electrophoresis and DNA sizing and sequencing. Each of the four molecules of DNA has a phosphate part that is negatively charged. When an electrical field is applied, DNA molecules move toward the positively charged anode. The size of DNA molecules can be measured when they are forced to migrate through a medium with different pore sizes, such as agarose or polyacrylamide gel. These gels serve as a molecular sieve to separate DNA molecules of different sizes. Gel electrophoresis is a widely used technique to size DNA molecules.

Sequencing is an application in which the relative order of the four nucleotides in a piece of DNA is determined. A sequencing procedure normally has two parts: biochemical reactions and gel electrophoresis. In the reactions, a series of DNA molecules with different size and fluorescent labeling is synthesized. When these products are separated in a sequencer, which uses gel electrophoresis to separate DNA fragments by size and by fluorescent color, the relative order of the four nucleotides of a DNA fragment can be determined. If we use a different reaction to produce a series of products in which the sizes represent alleles and the colors represent markers, the results obtained from the electrophoresis would be genotypes of the subject. This is the mechanism by which a DNA sequencer types microsatellites.

Allele-specific reactions for SNP typing. As described earlier, the alleles of SNP markers are defined by the nature of nucleotides at the polymorphic sites. Unlike microsatellite markers, different SNP marker alleles cannot be distinguished by the number of nucleotides or by the length of the molecules. For SNPs, determination of the alleles requires identifying which nucleotide occupies the polymorphic site. There are several ways to identify a nucleotide at a specific position; they rely on the properties of DNA polymerases and DNA ligases and on the physical properties of DNA molecules (Chen and Sullivan 2003; Kwok 2001; Syvanen 2001).

Genotyping Genetic Markers

VNTR markers. As shown in Figure 2–13A, the key characteristic of a VNTR marker is the tandem repeat of the same sequence motif. In the example shown, the motif is a CA dinucleotide. The variants or alleles of a VNTR marker are decided by the number of repeat units that a particular person has. So, to type a VNTR marker, we, in essence, count the number of repeats. A common protocol, therefore, includes a PCR to amplify the targeted locus and a gel electrophoresis to size the amplified fragments. To type a microsatellite marker, we design a pair of PCR primers to flank the repetitive sequence motif. Because the alleles of a microsatellite are defined by the number of repeats, subjects with different alleles will produce PCR products with different lengths. Using gel electrophoresis, we can differentiate the size of these PCR products. In other words, we can identify the alleles of the subjects.

SNP markers. The variants or alleles of a SNP marker are the bases at that particular location on the genome. The bases at the target site are identified by *SNP typing*. There are many methods of SNP typing, and they have been reviewed extensively (Chen and Sullivan 2003; Kwok 2001; Shi 2001; Syvanen 2001). Typically, genotyping protocols start with target amplification and follow with allelic discrimination and product detection/identification. In the allele-specific reactions, we explore the properties of DNA polymerases and ligases to identify the nucleotides at the polymorphic sites. In these reactions, only the presence of matching nucleotides produces allele-specific products. Because these products are generated only when the matching nucleotides exist, their identity reflects the alleles of the targets. The identification of these products, therefore, identifies the alleles of the subjects. With the technologies available today, investigators can genotype hundreds of thousands of targets a day.

Use of Other Measures in Linkage and Association Studies

The classical models of inherited (or "Mendelian") disorders, which are caused by alleles at one or two loci with very little environmental influence, do not apply to most complex psychiatric disorders. The number of genes may be large, their effects may be small, and their effects on the phenotype may be many and varied as a function of other contingencies, including those of chance and the environment. The identification of genes conferring susceptibility to psychiatric disorders requires approaches that do better justice to this complexity. No single, global method is likely to arise immediately. Studies will require ever more careful definition of the phenotype, by including other aspects of behavior and comorbid disorders that may reflect genetically different manifestations of the disease phenotype. It will be necessary to characterize the pathways from genes to outcome through better assessment of relevant endophenotypes. Recognition of the potential significance of developmental changes and genotype × environment interaction identifies the need for studies that combine careful assessment of both the phenotype and the environments that may alter the expression of genotypes that affect psychiatric disorders.

The search for smaller effects in systems for which the number of genetic and environmental contingencies is extremely large places a premium on sampling strategies and data-analytic methods that can minimize cost while also maximizing the proportion of reliable findings. This lesson was learned with classical twin studies in the 1970s and 1980s. Hand in hand with increased sophistication in the design of quantitative genetic studies was the development of more flexible and powerful methods of statistical analysis. As studies in psychiatric genetics focus on increasingly more outcomes, genes, and environments, the statistical landscape is expected to change again. Methods for the statistical analysis of large and complex data sets, such as neural network models and data-mining methods, are clearly headed in this direction, but it is still early and much remains to be done if the methods of genetic data analysis are to keep abreast of the enormous volume of data on genetic and environmental factors, which is likely to grow in the next few years.

Multiple Variables

Many of the designs and models described in this chapter are especially powerful when combined with the study of *multiple variables*. Most psychologists are familiar with two multivariate statistical methods: multiple regression and factor analysis. *Multiple regression* explores the relationships between *outcome variables*, such as depression, and *measured predictors*, such as age, sex and life events. Multiple regression models may include nonlinear functions of the measured variables in order to characterize hypothesized patterns of interaction between predictors. *Factor analysis* tries to account for the relationships between multiple outcomes in terms of one or more *latent variables* ("factors") whose effects have to be inferred from the relationships between measured variables. The classical example of a factor model is Spearman's (1904) model for the correlations between multiple abilities.

Multiple regression and factor analysis are special cases of a more general framework for exploring the underlying structure and relationships in multivariate data that has become known as *structural equation modeling* (e.g., Bollen 1989). In the 1960s and 1970s, Karl Jöreskog and his collaborators (see, e.g., Jöreskog 1978) developed methods to estimate the parameters of more general structural models and to test specific hypotheses about the number and contributions of latent variables to the patterns of association between multiple outcomes (*confirmatory factor analysis*). Figure 2–14 shows how Spearman's classical model for general and specific abilities can be represented in a path diagram.

Jöreskog and Sörbom (1996) developed LISREL (Linear Structural Relations) in the early 1970s as a first general program for structural equation modeling, and the program has subsequently evolved through several versions. Early genetic versions of structural equation modeling were implemented in LISREL (see Neale and Cardon 1992). Many recent developments have been aided

---

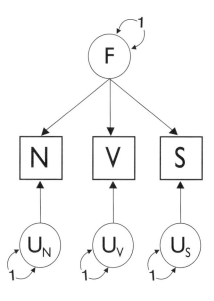

Figure 2–14. Path diagrammatic representation of a common factor model for differences in measured numerical (N), verbal (V), and spatial (S) abilities.

by more flexible software designed to meet some of the special challenges faced by genetic applications. Currently, the most flexible and widely used program in structural equation modeling of family data is Mx (Neale et al. 2004). Several other packages and programs for structural modeling display their own strengths and weaknesses. While these programs are capable of using a variety of statistical methods to fit models to the data, the most popular approach is to use the maximum likelihood framework.

In psychiatric genetics, structural equation modeling allows models for the effects of genes and environment in different kinds of family data to be extended to the multivariate case. Incorporation of genetically informative designs, such as the twin and adoption study in multivariate studies, may yield significant insight about the underlying causes of correlation between multiple measures.

Figure 2–15 shows how Spearman's (1904) classical factor model can be extended to take into account how genes and environment contribute to relationships between three variables in a classical

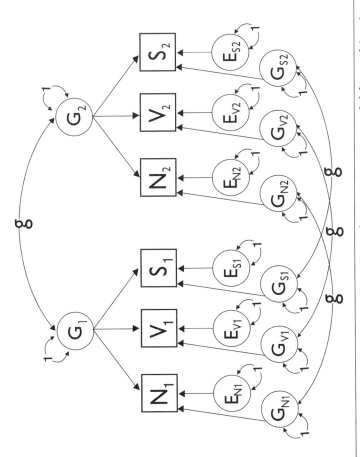

Figure 2–15. Illustrative extension of common factor to genetic model for multivariate twin data. See text for details.

twin study (see Martin and Eaves 1977). The effects of shared environment, *C*, are ignored for simplicity. The illustration assumes that each variable is affected by two kinds of genetic effect. Some of the variation is due to genes that affect all the outcomes ("general genetic factor"), and some of the variation in each measure is due to genes that affect that outcome only ("specific genetic effects"). In this case, the effects of the unique environment, *E*, are shown as purely trait-specific, although this is not required. The key to multivariate genetic analysis in twins is the information in cross-twin, cross-trait correlations—for example, the correlation between anxiety in one twin and depression in the co-twin. To the extent that anxiety and depression are influenced by the same genes, cross-twin, cross-trait correlations will be bigger in MZ than in DZ twins. Any correlation between traits may be caused partly by genes (the *genetic correlation*) and partly by the environment (the *environmental correlation*). Correlation *between* measures can be analyzed into its various genetic and environmental components just as we can analyze the variation *within* traits (e.g., Vandenberg 1965). There are now many examples of the multivariate genetic analysis of behavioral and psychiatric outcomes in twin studies. For example, Martin and Eaves (1977) found that the correlation between multiple measures of ability appeared to be genetic rather than environmental. Kendler et al. (1987) showed that symptoms of anxiety and depression had a strong underlying genetic communality but that separate environmental influences seemed to affect anxiety and depression. Silberg et al. (1996) concluded that there was, at least in part, a common genetic basis to variation in ADHD and antisocial behavior in adolescence. Such analyses provide a framework for understanding *comorbidity* of psychiatric disorders, since both genetic and environmental influences may create a phenotypic association between psychiatric outcomes (see Neale and Kendler 1995).

Applications of structural equation modeling continue to evolve. Models for other kinds of family data (adoptions, extensions of twin kinships) have been generalized to the multivariate case to account for assortative mating and nongenetic inheritance ("vertical cultural transmission"). Fulker (1988) summarized many of the conceptual issues at a more mathematical level. Structural equation modeling has been applied to the analysis of behavioral developmental models, multivariate genetic linkage (Eaves et al. 1997), and person-environment interplay. Extensions include application to categorical outcomes by means of the threshold model and item-response theory (IRT). Nonlinear structural equation models can allow for G×E interaction (see, e.g., Eaves et al. 2003; Kendler et al. 2003; Purcell and Sham 2002).

In the future, genotyping large numbers of markers, wider assessment of the environment, and increasing use of neuroimaging and microarray technology will generate enormous data sets with tens of thousands of variables. Such developments challenge statistical geneticists to develop still more flexible models and computational approaches to characterize the tortuous pathways from genes to complex behavioral phenotypes. Elements of many of these are now on the horizon with the development of computer-intensive data-mining methods, pattern recognition methods, and neural network models (see, e.g., Hastie et al. 2001 and York and Eaves 2001 for a genetic application).

The Developmental Process

The effects of genes on behavior are seldom expressed at birth but emerge during a dynamic developmental process involving both genes and social environment. The expression of differences at a later stage is contingent on preceding circumstances and is, to a greater or lesser extent, influenced by them. Thus, a full understanding of behavior and its disorders necessitates the analysis of the roles of genes and environment in development.

The unique value of longitudinal data for addressing questions of causality has long been realized. For example, if life events cause depression but not vice versa, we expect earlier life events to correlate with later depression more than we expect earlier depression to correlate with later life events. Such "cross-lagged" correlations are a powerful tool in the study of development, albeit one that should be interpreted with caution (see, e.g., Rogosa 1980). The power can often be enhanced still further when such designs are integrated with a genetically informative design, such as the longitudinal twin or adoption study. A more extended technical discussion of models for the genetic study of behavioral development is given by Neale et al. (2004). Here we try to distill some of the basic ideas.

The same approaches used to study behavior at a single time point extend naturally to the study of development. Usually, the study of development requires the repeated assessment of multiple behavioral outcomes and covariates such as parental treatment and life events. The combination of longitudinal data with a genetically informative design, such as the twin or adoption study, makes possible the behavior-genetic study of development. Several landmark longitudinal genetic studies are currently in progress, including the Louisville Twin Study (Wilson 1983); Minnesota Twin Family Study (Iacono and McGue 2002); Colorado Adoption Project (Plomin and DeFries 1985); Virginia Twin Study of Adolescent Behavioral Development (Eaves et al. 1997), and Missouri Twin Study (Heath et al. 2002). In addition, longitudinal twin studies exploring the role of genetic and environmental factors in the aging process are in progress (e.g., Pedersen et al. 1991).

At the conceptual level, the genetic analysis of development boils down to the analysis of multivariate genetic data in which separate occasions or ages of measurement constitute separate variables. Just as multivariate genetic analysis accounts for the patterns of genetic and environmental correlation between variables (see subsection "Multiple Variables" earlier in this chapter), so the analysis of development tries to explain patterns of genetic and environmental association over time. The inclusion of time, however, raises issues not normally considered in regular multivariate studies. First, although ages are often grouped for practical purposes (e.g., by age, by year of birth), time is really a continuous variable and needs to be treated as such in a developmental genetic analysis (Mehta and West 2000). Second, although the key to the genetic analysis of behavioral development lies in the patterns of covariance between measures over time, looking at the data in different ways—for example, by fitting individual growth curves—may yield a more economical and insightful explanation of the underlying process.

Approaches to the analysis of longitudinal genetic data fall into two groups. The *linear time-series* approach focuses on the pattern of covariance between repeated measures over time. Such models typically assume differences on a later occasion to depend partly on previous occasions ("continuity") and partly on new factors, genetic or environmental, that occur on each occasion ("innovation"). This basic model can be expressed in terms of both continuous and discrete time measures (Eaves et al. 1986). Time-series models for development often predict that 1) the variances and covariances between relatives increase with time to some stable value; 2) heritabilities may increase or decrease over time as a function of how the effects of genes and environment accumulate and decay with age; and 3) the genetic and/or environmental correlations between different ages tend to decay exponentially as a function of increasing age difference. The last-mentioned generates the so-called simplex structure to the matrices of cross-temporal correlations (Boomsma and Molenaar 1987). The simplex pattern arises because each age has its own novel genetic and environmental influences whose effects on subsequent occasions decline as new influences are constantly generated.

Figure 2–16 illustrates a possible form of a genetic time-series model and its implications for age changes in the contributions of genetic and environmental effects to variation in a trait measured over time. In the first version of the model, a single set of genetic differences (G) affects the phenotype directly at a series of repeated occasions (T_1–T_5 and onward) of measurement reflected in the single-headed arrow from G to each of T_1–T_5. In addition, each occasion has its own unique environmental effects (E_1–E_5). The particular feature of the time-series model is the pathway, b, between measurements at each time and the time immediately following. This pathway implies that effects persist and decay over time. These effects are equivalent to the influence of past experience on current behavior. For example, previous depression may create a greater risk for later depression. The fact that G affects behavior directly at each time implies that genetic risk to depression is a continuous factor in whether or not a person becomes depressed. A model that makes quite different predictions is obtained by deleting the dashed arrows from G to T_2–T_5 in Figure 2–16, leaving only the effects of genes at the start of the process ($T1$).

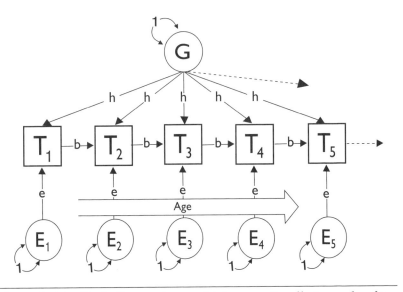

Figure 2–16. Basic time-series model for genetic effects on developmental change.
See text for details.

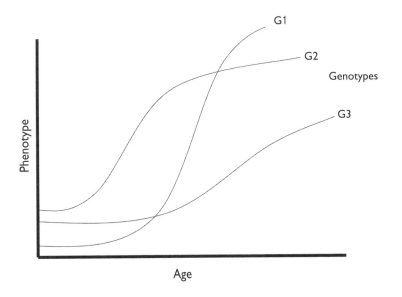

Figure 2–17. Simple growth curve model for genetic effects on developmental change.

Although this time-series approach has some conceptual strengths, the pattern of changes in mean and cross-temporal correlation may sometimes point to different and more parsimonious models for the developmental process. For example, the innovation/decay aspect of the time-series model cannot account adequately for the patterns of variance and covariance over time in the growth of plants or people. In such cases *growth curve models* may be better. They account for the patterns of temporal change in both mean and covariance, in terms of random genetic and/or environmental differences in the shape of the curves relating outcome to age. Such models are also known as *random regression models* or *hierarchial mixed models.* Individual differences in a linear growth process may result from genetic and environmental effects on starting value and/or rate of change. Other, nonlinear, curves may reflect differences in initial and final values and rates of change (see Figure 2–17). Curves with different mathematical properties may be appropriate in other circumstances (e.g., the time-dependent homeostatic response of the cardiovascular system to stress-induced perturbation; see Murphy and Trojak 1986). Underlying each of these basic kinds of model is an appreciation that individual differences in the parameters of change are accessible to the same kinds of genetic analysis (e.g., in terms of the multivariate ACE model in the case of repeated measures of MZ and DZ twins).

Although we speak of growth, the same conceptual approach may be used with any outcome that changes systematically over time. Figure 2–17 shows possible patterns of growth for three genetically different people, G_1, G_2, and G_3. The curves differ in initial and final phenotypes, the rate of growth, and the time of steepest growth. Each aspect of the growth process may have its own genetic control. Some of the genes may affect more than one process at the same time. For example, growth may be more rapid in individuals who start at the higher initial value. Past technical barriers to the full exploration of growth-curve models for longitudinal data are less applicable today (see Eaves et al. 2003; Neale and McArdle 2000), and there is increasing hope that the genetic analysis of longitudinal data may prove as flexible as any other aspect of behavior-genetic analysis. Neale et al. (2004) illustrate more general applications of the basic growth-curve approach to other systems (e.g., the dynamic adaptation of organisms to environmental stimuli).

Nature-Nurture Interplay: G×E Interaction

Genotype-environment correlation is characterized by genetic influences on *exposure* to the environment. By contrast, G×E (genotype × environment *interaction*) is characterized by genetic influences on *sensitivity* to the environment. G×E is a well-documented feature of genetic systems in experimental and commercial species from microorganisms through plants and fruit flies to mammals. Sensitivity to the environment is a trait like any other. Genetic variants affecting sensitivity to the environment can be manipulated by breeding and selection much as can any other aspect of the phenotype. The genes that control response to the environment are often different from those contributing to average response over a range of environments. That is, genes contributing to G×E can be separated from those contributing to the main effects of genes by breeding and selection.

Experimental studies have shown that in some cases different genes affect sensitivity to different features of the environment (e.g., temperature, rainfall, nutrients, maternal stress). In other cases, G¥E involves genes that respond to the integral of multiple features of the environment (i.e., to overall environmental quality). Genes may affect sensitivity to easily measured "macro-environmental" effects (e.g., temperature and rainfall) but also influence sensitivity to random, unmeasured "micro-environmental" effects.

When G×E is absent, the rate of response to changes in the environment is the same for every genotype (Figure 2–18A). In the presence of G×E, the slope of the response to the environment will vary according to genotype. In Figure 2–18B, the environment increases the phenotype for every genotype, but the rate of increase is greater for the genotypes with a higher mean value, increasing the genetic differences between people, but not their ranking, as the environment changes (this is known as *scalar G×E*).

Each gene may affect the average value of the phenotype over environments, sensitivity to the environment, or both. Figure 2–18C shows what is called *nonscalar G×E*, in which the ranking of genotypes changes with the environment. Mean effects of genotypes do not correlate with their slopes. The effect of G×E on the variances and correlations of relatives will depend on how the individual genes affect the location and slope of the response to differences in the environment. Figure 2–19A shows how the genetic variance of individuals changes with increasing environmental stress. Figure 2–19B shows a pattern of change expected in the genetic covariance between individuals measured in increasingly dissimilar environments under the two main types of G×E. Typically, detection of G×E requires measurement of the genotype (through genetic markers) or the environment, or both (see, e.g., Mather and Jinks 1982). However some genetically informative designs that include, for example, MZ and DZ twins, some of whom are reared in different homes, also permit detection of G×E from unspecified sources (Hershberger 2003; Jinks and Fulker 1970).

Attempts to analyze G×E by dividing samples by measured genotypes or environments require that genotypes and environments be independent (i.e., that there is no rGE) and that genes and environments be measured exactly so that they can be treated as fixed, known variables. This is unlikely to be the case for measures of the environment. Other models incorporate the analysis of G×E when the environments are not known perfectly and are correlated with genotype. The natural experiment of an adoption study provides a straightforward way to test for G×E interaction. In the case of a continuous phenotype, interaction may be detected with linear regression on 1) the mean of biological parents' phenotypes (which directly estimates heritability); 2) the mean of adoptive parents' phenotypes; and 3) the product of (1) and (2). Significance of the third term would indicate significant G×E interaction. With binary data such as psychiatric diagnoses, the rate in adoptees may be compared between subjects with biological or adoptive parents affected versus both affected. G×E interaction has been found for alcoholism (Cloninger et al. 1981) and substance abuse (Cloninger et al. 1985).

A

No GxE

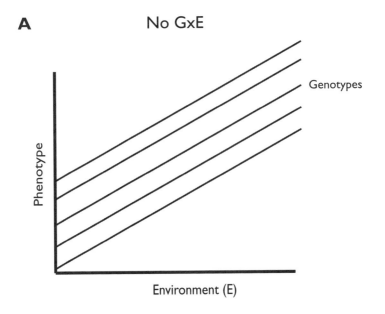

B

Scalar GxE

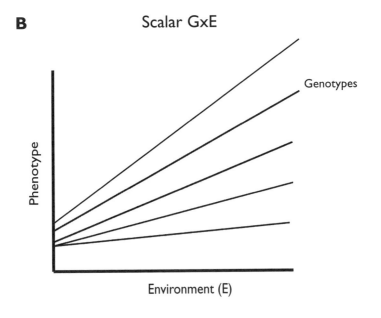

C Nonscalar GxE

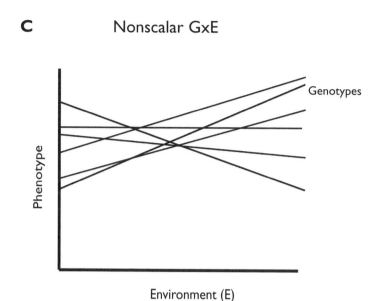

Figure 2–18. Sensitivity to the environment: additive model and examples of genotype × environment interaction (G×E). **(A)** No G×E. **(B)** Scalar G×E. **(C)** Nonscalar G×E.

Nature-Nurture Interplay: Genotype-Environment Correlation

Genotype-environment correlation (rGE) refers to a set of mechanisms in which genetic differences between individuals result in their being exposed to different, correlated environments. Christopher Jencks (1972) coined the term "double advantage" for one type of (positive) rGE in which children who are born with a genetic predisposition to high ability tend to create and experience more than an average share of stimulating environments. Genotype-environment correlation may arise as a direct function of individuals' own genotypes ("active" and "evocative" rGE) or as a secondary consequence of the social influence of people who are correlated with them genetically ("passive" rGE).

Figure 2–20 illustrates some of the pathways through which the different types of rGE may arise between parents and offspring.

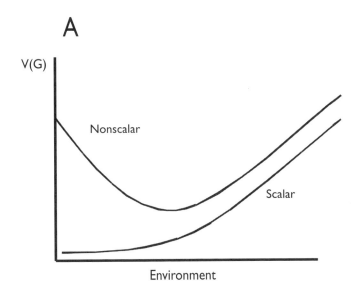

A

V(G)

Nonscalar

Scalar

Environment

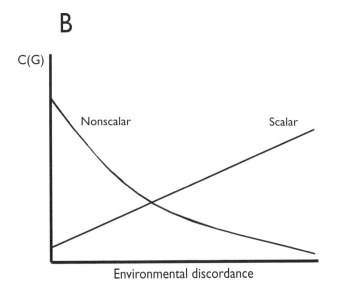

B

C(G)

Nonscalar

Scalar

Environmental discordance

Figure 2–19. Impact of additive and genotype x environment interaction (G×E) models for effects of genes and environment on genetic covariance between relatives as a function of difference in environment. **(A)** Genetic variance under G×E. **(B)** Genetic covariance under G×E.

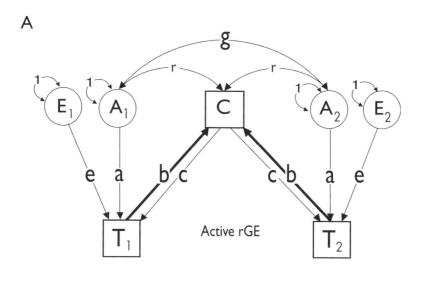

A

Active rGE

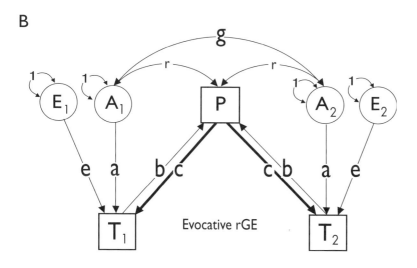

B

Evocative rGE

Figure 2–20. Genotype-environment correlation in parent-offspring interaction.

See text for details.

Genotype-environment correlation may arise because a person's own genes create or elicit the correlated environment. Robert Plomin and others distinguish between "active" and "evocative" rGE (e.g., Plomin and Bergman 1991; Plomin et al. 1977; Scarr and McCartney 1983). In the former case, individuals' own genetic constitutions make them choose or create nonrandom environments. Thus, genetic effects on smoking behavior would be a form of *active* rGE in the risk for cancer and coronary heart disease. *Evocative* rGE arises when the environment (typically other people) calibrates its response to individuals as a function of their genotypes. Both depend on the interplay between the individual and environment. Figures 2–20A and B illustrate active and evocative rGE between parents and twin children. An example of negative, evocative rGE is the tendency of parents and teachers to be more critical of children who show characteristics of (genetically influenced) antisocial behavior. Cattell (1963) coined the term "cultural coercion to the biosocial norm" to describe such evocative rGE.

Active rGE extends to the choice of social environment. Thus, there is growing evidence that genetic differences may influence the choice of friends (Iervolino et al. 2002). Equally important is the person-environment interplay that results in mate selection. Correlations between spouses are large and positive for many attitudinal and socioeconomic variables (Eaves et al. 1999). Typically, these correlations seem to result more from the active selection of spouses (*positive assortative mating*) than from reciprocal social influence of spouses. To the extent that genetic differences affect the traits involved in mate selection, assortative mating meets all the qualifications for active rGE. Positive assortative mating is a factor in establishing and maintaining social and genetic diversity while tending to limit social mobility between generations.

Active and evocative rGE warn against a simplistic reduction of genetic constructs to elementary genetic mechanisms. Jinks and Fulker (1970) noted that traditional estimates of heritability include all the correlated developmental consequences of early genetic differences. The term *person-environment interplay* underscores the fact that many genetic effects operate at a level far removed from the DNA. Once genes create a person, they create an organism that precipitates and interprets experience in ways that may reinforce—or counteract—primary genetic differences.

Critical to the understanding of rGE is the attempt to detect the effects of genes on putative environmental measures. Variations on the twin design can accomplish this goal. *Assessments of the twins' own environments* within the classical cross-sectional or longitudinal twin study permit the identification of active and evocative rGE. Such studies treat measures of the environment like any other aspect of the phenotype that may have a genetic component. Studies of this type have demonstrated that individual genetic differences may influence exposure to important life events (e.g., Kendler et al. 1993). *Multivariate genetic analysis* of psychiatric outcomes and environmental risk factors using the methods described above can be used to test alternative models of the roles of rGE in the relationship between specific environments, such as life events, and behavioral outcomes, such as depression. Including environmental assessments in a longitudinal genetic study may further enhance the resolution of active and evocative rGE. *Assessment of the environment twins provide for their children* (the children of twins, or COT, design described below) constitutes a powerful approach to the detection of passive rGE. The active correlation between the genotypes of twins and their behavior toward their children accounts for part of the passive rGE experienced by children.

What Is the Role of Environmental Indices in Twin Studies?

Figure 2–21 illustrates one conception of the parents of twins (POT) research design. The model is an extension of the ACE model (see Figure 2–9) in which the latent shared environmental effect (C) is replaced by the measured parental environment (P), affecting the phenotypes of the twins (T_1 and T_2). The design seeks to account for part of the shared environment in twin studies by referring to explicit features of the *measured environment*. Such measures are sometimes referred to as *environmental indices*. If environmental indices are pure measures of the environment, their correlation with the phenotype will be entirely environmental. Removing

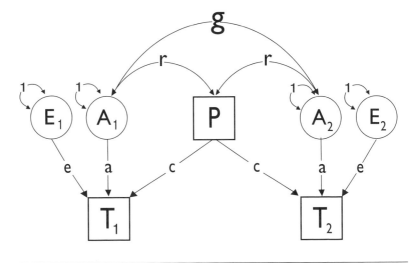

Figure 2–21. Twins and their parents: a possible conception. See text for explanation of variables.

the effects of such indices from the twins' phenotypes by regression will account for part of the variance due to the shared environment. However, the shared measured environment may also be correlated with the latent genetic effects on twins, so the assumption that there are no genetic effects on an environmental index may be misleading (see Meyer et al. 2000). This problem applies to attempts to measure both the home environment, because of passive rGE, and the environments of individuals, because of active and evocative rGE.

Do Parents Respond to Genetic Differences in Their Children?

We take it for granted that parents influence their children. However, children may also influence their parents; an old joke quips "Insanity is hereditary—you get it from your kids." That is, parental behavior is part of a child's extended phenotype and may be affected by genetic differences among children, which is an example of *evocative genotype-environment correlation*. If children affect parent-child interplay, then parents' treatment of MZ twins should be more similar than their treatment of DZ twins to the extent that parents are responding to differences in their children. An elegant early example of such a study was reported by Lytton (1977), who observed many facets of the interaction between parents and infant twin boys. Interactions in which parents took the initiative were equally correlated in MZ and DZ twins, whereas interactions in which parents responded to twins' behavior were more highly correlated in MZ twins. Studies by other investigators have shown that such evocative rGE is a fairly general feature of parent-child interaction. Figure 2–20, presented earlier in this chapter, illustrates one conception of the reciprocal interaction of parents and children.

What Do Parents Do to Their Children?

A growing series of studies in psychiatric genetics addresses the effects of parents on their children. Questions range from the effect of maternal smoking in pregnancy on offspring antisocial behavior to the effect of parental child-rearing behavior and attitudes on depression. Typical parent-offspring studies, including the POT study described in the previous section, can demonstrate an *association* between behavior in parents and their children but usually cannot identify its cause, because parents influence their children genetically as well as socially (see above). The *children of twins* (COT) design, with or without the extension to include the *spouses of twins* (C-SPOT), provides additional leverage on the causes of parent-offspring association (see, e.g., D'Onofrio et al. 2003; Heath and Eaves 1985; Heath et al. 1985; Silberg and Eaves 2004). As its name suggests, the valuable feature of the COT design is that many unique biological and social relationships can be derived from the study of twins and their children. Originally conceived of as the "MZ half-sib" design (Nance and Corey 1976), the approach focused on the children of identical twins as a new way of detecting the environmental effects of the maternal genotype on their children. Further extensions of the design and modeling have involved the inclusion of DZ twins and their children and exploited measures made on the twin parents as well as their children. A full model for the C-SPOT study tries to take into account a variety of additional factors, such as assortative mating.

Figure 2–22 illustrates a model for C-SPOT data. The measured variables are the phenotypes of the spouses, S_1 and S_2; the children, C_1 and C_2 of a pair of twins; and the phenotypes of the twins themselves, T_1 and T_2. The figure is an extension of a "three variable ACE model" in which the phenotypes of spouses and children are treated as aspects of the extended phenotypes of the twins themselves. Thus, there are genetic (GT), shared environmental (CT), and unique environmental (ET) effects that influence the phenotypes of the twins that also affect the phenotypes of spouses (through phenotypic assortment) and children (through genetic and nongenetic inheritance). Assortment may also be based on genes and environments (GS, CS, and ES) that affect choice of mates but not the phenotypes of the twins themselves. Finally, there may be additional child-specific genetic and environmental effects (GC, CC, and EC). GT, CT, and ET have a common influence on twins, spouses, and children. They explain the patterns of correlation between the twins themselves and any effect of the genes and environments of twins on the selection of spouses and the impact of twin parents on children. Note particularly that the path from ET to the children's phenotypes will be significant only if the behavior of the individual twins has a direct (environmental) effect on offspring behavior. GS and CS affect only spouses' phenotypes and reflect any additional genetic and shared environmental effects in the twins that affect choice of mate but not the phenotypes of twins. ES are any residual effects on spouses not explained by mate selection. The effect of ES on offspring phenotype explains any residual effects of spouses on children not explicable, directly or indirectly, through the effects of twins on mate selection and child behavior. The "child-specific" effects—GC, CC, and EC—all account for differences and correlations among the children of twins that cannot be accounted for by influences measured in the parents. The correlation between genetic effects in twins is $g = 1$ or $\frac{1}{2}$ in MZ and DZ twins, respectively. The residual genetic correlation between the children of twins (cousins related through MZ or DZ twins) is $\frac{1}{4}g$. Any genetic effects of assortative mating will be confounded by the various "shared environmental" parameters in this twin design, as in others.

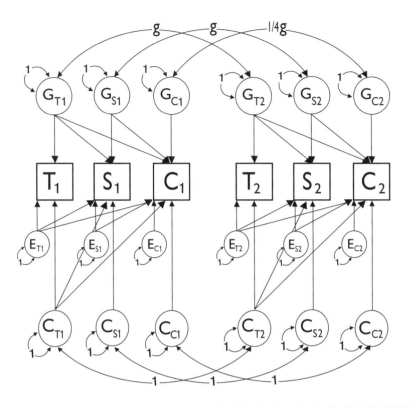

Figure 2–22. An "extended phenotype" model for twins and their spouses and children.
See text for details.

This brief discussion outlines some of the rich possibilities for understanding the processes of mate selection and family influence inherent in the C-SPOT design. The use of this design in psychiatric genetics is still in its infancy but has begun to attract attention from those seeking to resolve the genetic and environmental effects of parents on children.

Statistics: Estimating Effects and Testing a Model

What specific values of the model parameters best explain the observations?; How precisely are these values known? and Does the model fit the data? These questions form the core of model-fitting and parameter estimation. No model is expected to fit all data sets perfectly, but some models may fit better than others. Every model involves a number of "free parameters," that is, quantities such as path coefficients that are unknown but are to be estimated from the data. For a given model, one approach to estimation is to search for parameter values that give the best possible fit to observed correlations, means, variances, and co-variances between relatives. *Goodness-of-fit* is judged by a mathematical function, the so-called loss function, that measures the discrepancy between the observed data and the values predicted from the model. The best loss functions have known statistical properties so that observed discrepancies in fit can be compared with those expected by chance alone.

Ronald Fisher introduced the concept of likelihood that is widely used as a guide to comparing models in psychiatric genetics (Edwards 1972). Models that fit very poorly are less likely to have generated the observations in question than models that fit well. Within a given model, different parameter values are more or less likely to have generated the specific data of interest. Intuitively, the best estimates of model parameters are those that *maximize the likelihood* of the data.

Among models that fit adequately, other selection criteria, such as relative simplicity (i.e., having fewer parameters) or coherence within a broader theoretical framework and other data, may be used as well. A variety of automated computational methods, or *numerical optimizers,* have been developed that search for maximum-likelihood parameter estimates (see, e.g., Neale and Cardon 1992).

Power

Fifty years ago, the main question being asked was whether a particular behavioral trait had a genetic component, and a study with a sample of 100 twin pairs was considered large. By the 1970s, questions were more subtle, and the samples grew to several hundred or even a thousand pairs. By the 1980s and 1990s, researchers were looking for samples of several thousand. At the heart of this change was a growing concern for statistical power. Typically, the effects of chance decrease as samples get relatively larger so conclusions get more precise and more trustworthy. The concept of *power* provides a quantitative framework for answering such questions as "Will my study be big enough to find a gene at this location?" or "Can I hope to detect a shared environmental effect with this number of twin pairs?" Consideration of power is critical to planning any new study.

Evaluation of power in genetic studies usually requires calculations that are most easily done on a computer, though simpler calculations often give an approximate estimate. The power of a study will depend on the question being asked, the hypothesized size of the effect of interest, the design of the study, the method of statistical analysis, and the significance level used to choose between hypotheses. Every power calculation requires that these factors be specified.

Figure 2–23 illustrates the analysis of power for a linkage study as the amount of variance due to a QTL changes in an unselected sample of sib pairs. As can be seen in the figure, a total sample of 1,294 pairs would have to be measured and genotyped to achieve 80% power at the 5% significance level if the QTL explains 20% of the variance. If we are interested in a QTL that explains only 10% of the variance (still quite a "big" gene), the sample size is quite prohibitively large (5,205 pairs). These number of pairs increases considerably once the required significance level is increased to control for multiple testing that is inevitable in a genome scan.

In practice, power in a linkage study depends on several additional factors: the distance between Q and M, and the degree of polymorphism in the marker. The power decreases as the distance increases and when M is not highly polymorphic. Increasing the sample size increases power by increasing how much we know about the correlations. Results of a power analysis are both hypothesis-specific and design-specific. In the case represented in Figure 2–23, we assumed that we were going to test for linkage at a single location on the genome, using a random sample of sib pairs. We would get a different answer if we were to use a *sample selected for specific criteria*. Examples of such approaches are the affected sib

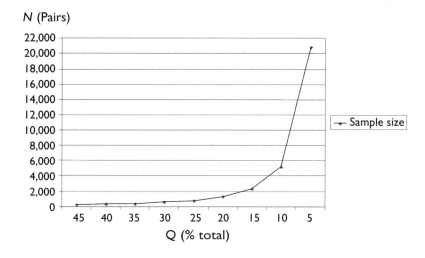

Figure 2–23. Illustration of power calculations applied to design of a linkage study.
Number of pairs needed to obtain 80% power to detect QTL effect contributing different proportions (Q) of the total variance.

pair design, or the discordant sib pair design, or some judicious combination of both (see, e.g., Risch and Zhang 1995) selected from a much larger population of random sibling pairs. Analysis of such selected samples requires statistical approaches that make appropriate allowance for missing data (Little and Rubin 1987).

The same concept applies to the design of other studies in genetic epidemiology. No single study is best for every purpose. In general, study design requires a balance of judgment between optimizing a design to focus powerfully on one or two specific questions and designing a study to test a broader range of hypotheses, perhaps with somewhat reduced power. Studies designed to test for interactions (e.g., between the effects of genes and covariates such as sex or aspects of the social environment) typically require much larger samples than studies designed to identify main effects.

The above discussion is based on testing individual hypotheses specified in advance. Exploratory studies, such as those designed to analyze many different outcomes, and studies designed to search large regions of the genome (i.e., very many genetic markers) for evidence of linkage or association will almost certainly require larger samples. As the number of statistical tests mounts, so does the chance of false positive findings. Sham (1997) provides a more detailed consideration of these issues in relation to linkage studies. Multistage designs—in which large numbers of outcomes or risk factors are screened initially, on the basis of relatively liberal criteria for significance, as a prelude to selecting variables (e.g., loci) that can be subjected to more extensive scrutiny—offer one cost-effective approach to such exploratory studies.

Conclusion

The behavioral phenotype is far removed from the primary effects of genes. To arrive at a comprehensive understanding of how genes influence complex behavioral disorders, psychiatric geneticists have to grapple with a series of questions about how the effects of genes are translated through development via the interplay of genes and environment. No single approach can answer every question. The tools available to the psychiatric geneticist are evolving rapidly. Each new technological development in molecular biology and the neurosciences poses new opportunities and challenges for the design and analysis of genetic studies. Soon, perhaps, it will be cost effective to characterize variation and expression at most, if not all, genes. Techniques for visualizing the structure and function of the brain are evolving rapidly. Such technical capabilities inspire different approaches to data collection and statistical analysis that are already being anticipated in advance of the data.

Questions about the intricate pathways and interactions of genes and environment remain that will challenge the ingenuity of the next generation of researchers. Older and newer models and methods will need to be integrated by investigators from many disciplines working together to provide the insights that may ultimately yield a comprehensive understanding of human behavior and its disorders.

References

Allison DB, Neale MC: Joint tests of linkage and association for quantitative traits. Theor Popul Biol 60:239–251, 2002

Bollen KA: Structural Equations With Latent Variables. New York, Wiley, 1989

Boomsma DI, Molenaar PCM: The genetic analysis of repeated measures. Behav Genet 17:111–123, 1987

Cadoret RJ: Psychopathology in adopted-away offspring of biologic parents with antisocial behavior. Arch Gen Psychiatry 35:176–184, 1978

Cadoret RJ, Troughton E, O'Gorman TW, et al: An adoption study of genetic and environmental factors in drug abuse. Arch Gen Psychiatry 43:1131–1136, 1986

Cardon LR, Abecasis GR: Using haplotype blocks to map human complex trait loci. Trends Genet 19:135–140, 2003

Carey G: Sibling imitation and contrast effects. Behav Genet 16:319–341, 1986

Cattell RB: The interaction of heredity and environmental influences. British Journal of Statistical Psychology 16:191–210, 1963

Chen X, Sullivan PF: Single nucleotide polymorphism genotyping: biochemistry, protocol, cost and throughput. Pharmacogenomics J 3:77–96, 2003

Cloninger CR, Bohman M, Sigvardsson S: Inheritance of alcohol abuse: cross-fostering analysis of adopted men. Arch Gen Psychiatry 38:861–868, 1981

Cloninger CR, Bohman M, Sigvardsson S, et al: Psychopathology in adopted-out children of alcoholics: The Stockholm Adoption Study, in Recent Developments in Alcoholism, Vol 3. Edited by Galanter M. New York, Plenum, 1985, pp 37–51

Dawkins R: The Extended Phenotype: The Gene as the Unit of Selection. Oxford, England, Oxford University Press, 1982

D'Onofrio BM, Turkheimer EN, Eaves LJ, et al: The role of the children of twins design in elucidating causal relations between parent characteristics and child outcomes. J Child Psychol Psychiatry 44:1130–1144, 2003

Eaves LJ: A model for sibling effects in man. Heredity 35:206–214, 1976

Eaves LJ, Erkanli A: Markov Chain Monte Carlo approaches to analysis of genetic and environmental components of human developmental change and G×E interaction. Behav Genet 33:279–299, 2003

Eaves LJ, Silberg JL: Parent-child feedback predicts sibling contrast: using twin studies to test theories of parent-offspring interaction in infant behavior. Twin Res (in press)

Eaves LJ, Last KA, Young PA, et al: Model-fitting approaches to the analysis of human behavior. Heredity 41:249–320, 1978

Eaves LJ, Long J, Heath AC: A theory of developmental change in quantitative phenotypes applied to cognitive development. Behav Genet 16:143–162, 1986

Eaves LJ, Silberg JL, Meyer JM, et al: The main effects of genes and environment on major behavioral problems of adolescence in the Virginia Twin Study of Adolescent Behavioral Development. J Child Psychol Psychiatry 38:965–980, 1997

Eaves LJ, Heath AC, Martin N, et al: Comparing the biological and cultural inheritance of personality and social attitiudes in the Virginia 30,000 study of twins and their relatives. Twin Res 2:62–80, 1999

Eaves LJ, Silberg JL, Erkanli AL: Resolving multiple epigenetic pathways to adolescent depression. J Child Psychol Psychiatry 44:1006–1014, 2003

Edwards AWF: Likelihood. London, Cambridge University Press, 1972

Ewens WJ, Spielman RS: The transmission/disequilibrium test: history, subdivision, and admixture. Am J Hum Genet 57:455–464, 1995

Falconer DF: The inheritance of liability to certain diseases, estimated from the incidence among relatives. Ann Hum Genet 29:51–76, 1965

Falconer DS, Mackay TFC: Introduction to Quantitative Genetics, 4th Edition. New York, Pearson Prentice Hall, 1996

Feldman MW, Lewontin RC: The heritability hang-up. Science 190:1163–1168, 1975

Ferreira MAR: Linkage analysis: principles and methods for the analysis of human quantitative traits. Twin Res 7:513–530, 2004

Fisher RA: The correlation between relatives on the supposition of Mendelian inheritance. Transactions of the Royal Society of Edinburgh 52:399–433, 1918

Fulker DW: Genetic and cultural transmission in human behavior, in Proceedings of the Second International Conference on Quantitative Genetics. Edited by Weir BS, Eisen EJ, Goodman MM, et al. Sunderland, MA, Sinauer, 1988, pp 318–340

Fulker DW, Cherny SS, Sham PC, et al: Combined linkage and association sib pair analysis for quantitative traits. Am J Hum Genet 64:259–267, 1999

Galton F: Hereditary Genius: An Inquiry Into Its Laws and Consequences. London, MacMillan, 1869

Galton F: Inquiries Into Human Faculty and Its Development. New York, AMS Press, 1883

Haseman KJ, Elston RC: The investigation of linkage between a quantitative trait and a marker locus. Behav Genet 2:3–19, 1972

Hasler G, Drevets WC, Manji HK, et al: Discovering endophenotypes for major depression. Neuropsychopharmacology 29:1765–1781, 2004

Hastie T, Tibshirani R, Friedman J: The Elements of Statistical Learning: Data Mining, Inference and Prediction. New York, Springer, 2001

Heath AC, Eaves LJ: Resolving the effects of phenotype and social background on mate selection. Behav Genet 15:15–30, 1985

Heath AC, Kendler KS, Eaves LJ, et al: The resolution of biological and cultural inheritance: the informativeness of different relationships. Behav Genet 15:439–465, 1985

Heath AC, Howells W, Bucholz KK, et al: Ascertainment of a midwestern US female adolescent twin cohort for alcohol studies: assessment of sample representativeness using birth record data. Twin Res 5: 107–112, 2002

Hershberger SL: Latent variable models of genotype-environment covariance. Structural Equation Modeling: A Multidisciplinary Journal. 10:423–434, 2003

Heston LL: Psychiatric disorders in foster home reared children of schizophrenic mothers. Br J Psychiatry 112:819–825, 1966

Iacono WG, McGue M: Minnesota Twin Family Study. Twin Res 5:482–487, 2002

Iervolino AC, Pike A, Manke B, et al: Genetic and environmental influences in adolescent peer socialization: evidence from two genetically sensitive designs. Child Dev 73:162–174, 2002

Jencks C: Inequality: A Reassessment of the Effects of Family and Schooling in America. New York, Basic Books, 1972

Jinks JL, Fulker DW: Comparison of the biometrical, genetical, MAVA and classical approaches to the analysis of human behavior. Psychol Bull 73:311–349, 1970

Jöreskog KG: Structural analysis of covariance and correlation matrices. Psychometrika 43:443–477, 1978

Jöreskog KG, Sörbom D: LISREL 8 User's Reference Guide. Chicago, IL, Scientific Software International, 1996

Kaprio J, Koskenvuo M, Langinvainio H: Finnish twins reared apart: smoking and drinking habits. Preliminary analysis of the effect of heredity and environment. Acta Genet Med Gemellol (Roma) 33:425–433, 1984

Kendler KS, Heath AC, Martin NG, et al: Symptoms of anxiety and symptoms of depression: same genes, different environments? Arch Gen Psychiatry 44:451–457, 1987

Kendler KS, Neale MC, Kessler RC, et al: A twin study of recent life events and difficulties. Archives of General Psychiatry 50:789–796, 1993

Kendler KS, Aggen SH, Jacobson KC, et al: Does the level of family dysfunction moderate the impact of genetic factors on the personality trait of neuroticism? Psychol Med 33:817–825, 2003

Kety SS: The significance of genetic factors in the etiology of schizophrenia: results from the National Study of Adoptees in Denmark. J Psychiatr Res 21:423–429, 1987

Kruglyak L, Lander ES: Complete multipoint sib-pair analysis of qualitative and quantitative traits. Am J Hum Genet 57:439–454, 1995

Kwok PY: Methods for genotyping single nucleotide polymorphisms. Annu.Rev Genomics Hum Genet 2:235–258, 2001

Little RJA, Rubin DB: Statistical Analysis With Missing Data. New York, Wiley, 1987

Lytton H: Do parents create or respond to differences in twins? Dev Psychol 13:456–459, 1977

Martin NG, Eaves LJ: The genetical analysis of covariance structure. Heredity 38:79–95, 1977

Mather K, Jinks JL: Biometrical Genetics: The Study of Continuous Variation. London, Chapman Hall, 1982

Mehta PD, West SG: Putting the individual back into growth curves. Psychol Methods 5:23–43, 2000

Mendel G: Experiments in plant hybridization (1866), in Principles of Genetics. Edited by Sinnott EW, Dunn LC, Dobzhansky T. New York, McGraw Hill, 1958, pp 419–443

Meyer JM, Rutter ML, Silberg JL, et al: Familial aggregation for conduct disorder symptomatology: the role of genes, marital discord, and family adaptability. Psychol Med 30:759–774, 2000

Morton NE: Analysis of family resemblance, I: introduction. Am J Hum Genet 26:318–330, 1974

Murphy EA, Trojak JL: The genetics of quantifiable homeostasis, I: the general issues. Am J Med Genet 24:159–169, 1986

Nance WE, Corey LA: Genetic models for the analysis of data from the families of identical twins. Genetics 83:811–826, 1976

Neale MC: The use of Mx for association and linkage analysis. Genescreen 1:107–111, 2001

Neale MC, Cardon LR: Methodology for Genetic Studies of Twins and Families. Dordrecht, Kluwer Academic, 1992

Neale MC, Kendler KS: Models of comorbidity for multifactorial disorders. Am J Hum Genet 57:935–953, 1995

Neale MC, McArdle JJ: Structured latent growth curves for twin data. Twin Res 3:165–177, 2000

Neale MC, Boker SM, Xie G, et al: Mx: Statistical Modeling. Richmond, Virginia Institute for Psychiatric and Behavioral Genetics, 2004

Ott J: Analysis of Human Genetic Linkage. Baltimore, MD, Johns Hopkins University Press, 1999

Pearson K: On the correlations of characters not quantitatively measurable. Philosophical Transactions of the Royal Society of London A 195:1–47, 1900

Pearson K: On the laws of inheritance in man, II: on the inheritance of the mental and moral characters in man, and its comparison with the inheritance of the physical characters. Biometrika 3:131–190, 1904

Pearson K, Lee A: On the laws of inheritance in man. Biometrika 2:356–462, 1903

Pedersen NL, McClearn GE, Plomin R, et al: The Swedish Adoption Twin Study of Aging: an update. Acta Genet Med Gemellol (Roma) 40:7–20, 1991

Plomin R, Bergman CS: The nature of nurture: genetic influence on "environmental" measures. Behav Brain Sci 14:373–386, 1991

Plomin R, DeFries JC: Origins of Individual Differences in Infancy: The Colorado Adoption Project. Orlando, FL, Academic Press, 1985

Plomin R, DeFries JC, Loehlin JC: Genotype-environment interaction and correlation in the analysis of human behavior. Psychol Bull 84:309–322, 1977

Purcell S, Sham P: Variance components models for gene-environment interaction in twin analysis. Twin Res 5:554–571, 2002

Rice J, Cloninger CR, Reich T: Multifactorial inheritance with cultural transmission and assortative mating, I: description and basic properties of unitary models. Am J Hum Genet 30:618–643, 1978

Risch N, Zhang H: Extreme discordant sib pairs for mapping quantitative trait loci in humans. Science 268:1584–1589, 1995

Rogosa DA: A critique of cross-lagged correlation. Psychol Bull 88:245–258, 1980

Rutter ML, Silberg JL: Gene-environment interplay in relation to emotional and behavioral disturbance. Ann Rev Psychol 53:463–490, 2001

Scarr S, McCartney K: How people make their own environments: a theory of genotype-environment effects. Child Dev 54:424–435, 1983

Schumaker RE, Marcoulides GE: Interaction and Nonlinear Effects in Structural Equation Modeling. Mahwah, NJ, Erlbaum, 1998

Sham P: Statistics in Human Genetics. London, Arnold, 1997

Shastry BS: SNPs and haplotypes: genetic markers for disease and drug response (review). Int J Mol Med 11:379–382, 2003

Shi MM: Enabling large-scale pharmacogenetic studies by high-throughput mutation detection and genotyping technologies. Clin Chem 47:164–172, 2001

Silberg JL, Eaves LJ: Analysing the contributions of genes and parent-child interaction to childhood behavioural and emotional problems: a model for the children of twins. Psychol Med 34:347–356, 2004

Silberg JL, Rutter ML: Nature-nurture interplay in the risks associated with parental mental disorder, in Children of Depressed Parents: Alternative Pathways to Risk for Psychopathology. Edited by Goodman S. New York, Wiley, 2001

Silberg JL, Rutter ML, Meyer JM, et al: Genetic and environmental influences on the covariation between hyperactivity and conduct disturbance in juvenile twins. J Child Psychol Psychiatry 37:803–816, 1996

Sorensen TI: The genetics of obesity. Metabolism 44:4–6, 1995

Spearman C: "General intelligence": objectively determined and measured. Am J Psychol 15:201–293, 1904

Syvanen AC: Accessing genetic variation: genotyping single nucleotide polymorphisms. Nat Rev Genet 2:930–942, 2001

Thomas DC: Statistical Methods in Genetic Epidemiology. Oxford, England, Oxford University Press, 2004

Truett KR, Eaves LJ, Walkers EE, et al: A model system for analysis of family resemblance in extended kinships of twins. Behav Genet 24:35–49, 1994

Vandenberg SG: Multivariate analysis of twin differences, in Methods and Goals in Human Behavior Genetics. Edited by Vandenberg SG. New York, Academic Press, 1965, pp 29–43

Weber JL, Broman KW: Genotyping for human whole-genome scans: past, present, and future. Adv Genet 42:77–96, 2001

Wilson RS: The Louisville Twin Study: developmental synchronies in behavior. Child Dev 54:298–316, 1983

Wright S: Correlation and causation. Journal of Agricultural Research 20:557–585, 1921

York TP, Eaves LJ: Common disease analysis using Multivariate Adaptive Regression Splines (MARS): Genetic Analysis Workshop 12 simulated sequence data. Genet Epidemiol 21 (suppl 1):S649–S654, 2001

Chapter 3

Genetics of Schizophrenia

Linkage and Association Studies

Brien Riley, Ph.D.
Kenneth S. Kendler, M.D.

The current model of liability to schizophrenia holds that both genetic and environmental risk factors contribute to the development of the illness. Although no risk factor of either type has yet been unambiguously identified, recent progress suggests that we are closer to understanding specific genetic influences than we are to characterizing specific environmental ones. To understand why this is so and to lay the foundation for discussing the interplay of genetic and environmental factors in schizophrenia, we review here what is known about the genetics of schizophrenia in some detail. Throughout this review, we also consider how this field of study continues to inform our understanding of the potential structure of environmental risk factors.

Genetic study of any complex trait, including schizophrenia, is based on and understood through two key areas of inquiry. First, genetic epidemiology asks whether there is additional risk for a trait in the relatives of cases and, if so, whether the risk is attributable to shared genetic versus shared environmental factors. The answers to these questions explain why we are looking for schizophrenia liability genes and what we think we might find. Second, association and linkage studies ask, respectively, whether there is a relationship between a trait and specific genes or between a trait and specific regions of the genome. An understanding of the underlying causes of these two genetic phenomena, the methods for detecting them, and the limitations of each is essential for a critical assessment of the evidence. The enormous amount of linkage and association data must be assessed in light of the two conceptual areas above to determine where the evidence is best that a liability gene occurs. In this chapter, we provide a broad overview of these concepts, integrating the results of many studies, and discuss the most promising current areas of investigation and insights from contemporary practitioners.

Genetic Epidemiology: Why Look for Genes That Contribute to Schizophrenia?

A large body of data collected from families, twins, and adoptees over many years has consistently supported the involvement of a major, complex genetic component in liability to schizophrenia and schizophrenia spectrum disorders.

Family Studies: Does Risk Aggregate in Relatives?

The combined results of the major European family studies published between 1921 and 1987 (Gottesman 1991) are shown in Figure 3–1. The lifetime morbid risk (MR) of schizophrenia is about 1% in the general population, but approximately 10 times that in the siblings or offspring of patients with schizophrenia. Smaller but consistent increases in MR are seen in second- and third-degree relatives. Criticisms of the methodology of early family studies included lack of proper controls, nonsystematic methods of sampling, lack of standardized diagnostic criteria, and failure to diagnose family members while blind to the status of the index case patient (or proband). A combined analysis of data from 7 studies that avoided these weaknesses yielded totals of 15 cases of schizophrenia in 3,035 lifetimes at risk in the control families, and 116 cases of schizophrenia in 2,418 lifetimes at risk in the patient families. These data translate into an average MR for narrowly defined schizophrenia of 0.5% for relatives of controls and 4.8% for relatives of patients with schizophrenia (Kendler and Diehl 1993). In other words, the more recent, methodologically stronger studies replicated the finding from earlier studies that a close relative of a schizophrenia patient has, on average, 10 times the baseline population risk of developing the disorder.

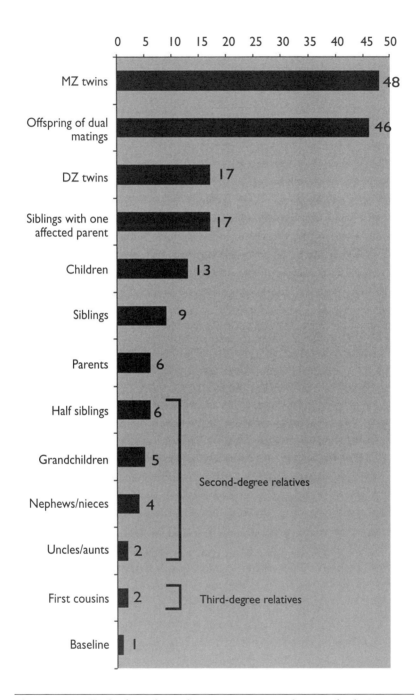

Figure 3–1. Risks for schizophrenia in various classes of relatives.

Twin Studies: How Large Is the Genetic Component of Risk?

Studies of twins provide a way to estimate the relative importance of shared genetic material and shared environment in the development of a trait. Twin studies of schizophrenia have been reviewed in detail by Cardno and Gottesman (2000). These studies show consistent evidence of a genetic effect, with higher concordance in monozygotic (~50%) than in dizygotic (~17%) twins. Both individual twin studies (Cardno et al. 1999; Farmer et al. 1987) and meta-analyses of twin studies (Sullivan et al. 2003) estimate the heritability of liability to schizophrenia to be approximately 80%. Sullivan et al. (2003), in their meta-analysis also found evidence that a small proportion of liability to schizophrenia (~11% of the total) resulted from shared environmental risk factors. Studies of twins show clearly that liability to schizophrenia is largely genetically *mediated,* but not genetically *determined,* and is thus a *complex* trait, determined by genes, environment, and their interaction.

Adoption Studies: Is Familial Aggregation Due to Shared Environment?

Across all adoption studies performed, the increased risk of schizophrenia is present in the biological relatives of patients with schizophrenia (Prescott and Gottesman 1993). The first adoption study found that 5 of 47 adopted-away offspring (16.6%) of schizophrenic mothers had schizophrenia compared with 0 of 50 adopted-away offspring of control mothers (Heston 1966). In Finland, a much larger study of adopted-away offspring of schizophrenic mothers found that in 361 families of adopted offspring, 13 of the 144 children (9.1%) of schizophrenic mothers had a schizophrenia spectrum disorder and 7 of 144 (4.9%) had schizophrenia, whereas only 2 of the 178 control offspring (1.1%) had schizophrenia (Tienari 1991). In studies of adoptees in Denmark, schizophrenia was found to be significantly more common in the biological relatives of schizophrenic adoptees than in the biological relatives of control adoptees in both urban and nonurban samples (Kety et al. 1968, 1994). The rates of schizophrenia were low and not different in the adoptive families of both affected and control groups.

Segregation Analysis: How Is the Genetic Risk Transmitted?

Transmission models are mathematical expressions of a hypothetical genetic architecture for a trait and allow us to make specific predictions about risk in various classes of relatives. Such models are tested by assessing how well their predictions match observed patterns of risk. The risk patterns for single-gene disorders are expressed by means of the generalized *single major locus* (SML) model, which assumes that a single gene is responsible for all liability. These two terms, *gene* and *locus,* are often used interchangeably, though they have specific meanings. A *locus* is simply a position on a chromosome (e.g., a place where linkage or association is observed) that may or may not represent a *gene,* the specific DNA template for a polypeptide or functional RNA unit.

Studies of the patterns of risk for schizophrenia in relatives generally conclude that the familial transmission of schizophrenia cannot be explained solely by a single gene. The *multifactorial threshold* (MT) model is less genetically deterministic; it assumes instead a continuum of liability due to multiple genetic and environmental factors, in the upper reaches of which, a person has a high risk of developing schizophrenia. An analysis of the data from a carefully selected number of European studies demonstrated that neither the SML nor the MT model is adequate to explain observed patterns of risk (McGue et al. 1985).

Although these results seem to bring us no closer to a model with good predictive power, they both suggest a conclusion with far-reaching consequences for molecular genetic research: that the genetic liability for schizophrenia is, at least in part, transmitted by multiple interacting (or *epistatic*) genes. The MT model, which has great intuitive appeal but poor predictive power, assumes that the effects of multiple genes on risk combine *additively* (the total liability from *n* genes is *equal* to the sum of the *n* individual liabilities) and that there are no interactions among them. A key predictive failure of the MT model is that the observed concordance rate in monozygotic twins (~50%) is too high relative to the risk in siblings and dizygotic twins (9%–17%). Such a pattern is more consistent with involvement of multiple epistatic genes, in which the total liability from n genes is *greater than* the sum of the n individual liabilities, and gene-gene or gene-environment interactions. The falloff in concordance rates for schizophrenia in first-, second-, and third-degree relatives in the families of patients with schizophrenia found in a study by Risch (1990) is also most consistent with multiple epistatically interacting genes, although that study did not model the impact of reduced fertility (which is large in individuals with schizophrenia), which could have introduced a substantial source of bias in the results. Basic modeling with minimal assumptions shows that as the number of such genes increases, the risk-bearing alleles at these loci become very common in the population (on the order of 14%–20%) (Riley et al. 1997).

Conversely, if the inheritance model was fully epistatic, then the *tetrachoric correlation* (the correlation in the normally distributed liability to illness) in MZ twins should be substantially more than twice that seen in DZ twins, which is not observed. Additionally, recent studies have suggested that *genetic × environment interactions* (G×Es) are important components of the overall risk for conduct disorder (Caspi et al. 2002; Foley et al. 2004) and depression (Caspi et al. 2003; Kendler et al., in press), and possibly for schizophrenia as well (Tienari et al. 2004; see also Kendler et al., in press).

Although segregation analyses have not provided a definitive inheritance model for the genetic risk for schizophrenia, it is probably safe to conclude that numerous kinds of influences (including both additive and epistatic genetic factors as well as G×Es) are involved. Segregation analyses of a single complex model, such as the MT model or the epistatic model, are already extremely difficult. Analysis of a multiple-component model, such as the one we suggest above, will be even more difficult, and it seems unlikely that a definitive model for the inheritance of genetic liability to schizophrenia will be developed prior to understanding a significant number of the genes involved and their interactions.

Epistatically interacting genes will show smaller effects when examined singly than will those that combine additively, since the proportion of total risk associated with a single gene in an epistatic system is less than that for a single gene in an additive system with the same n genes. Interacting genes must also be biologically related—functionally and temporally or spatially. Epistatic interaction is only possible if the *genotype* (the pair of *alleles,* or variable forms, of a gene present in a normal human chromosome complement) or *phenotype* (the observable effect of that genotype) from one gene exerts an effect on the phenotype from another. It follows from this that environmental risk factors that interact with the genetic vulnerabilities must also be biologically related (functionally, temporally or spatially) to them, though other kinds of environmental risk factors that do not interact with genetic vulnerabilities are also possible. Modeling such synergistic interaction for hypothesis testing or data analysis is much more complex than modeling additive combination, since the risk for particular genotypes (also called *penetrance*) at different loci must be defined, and this requires specifying the genes and genotypes, and their contribution, a priori. At our current stage of research on most complex genetic traits, in which the individual genes contributing to risk are unknown, this is not possible.

Spectrum Disorders: How Broad Is the Range of Psychiatric Illness Transmitted, and Who Is Affected?

Kendler and Diehl (1993) reviewed results from studies of illnesses other than schizophrenia in relatives of schizophrenia patients. Again, only studies that used rigorous methodology, including personal interviews, structured diagnostic criteria, and blind diagnoses, were considered. The results are extremely variable across studies and different conditions examined. In five of seven studies, the risk of schizotypal personality disorder (SPD) or paranoid personality disorder (PPD) in relatives of patients with schizophrenia was consistent, at 4–4.5 times that in the control families. Of seven studies (overlapping those above) that met the same criteria and examined the risk of schizoaffective, schizophreniform, and delusional disorders, and atypical psychosis in the relatives of patients, five showed significantly higher risks of these conditions, as well. Two other studies, examining the converse of the question, found that the risk of schizophrenia is significantly higher in the relatives of individuals with schizoaffective disorder and schizophreniform disorder than in controls (Kendler et al. 1986, 1993).

Studies of wider spectra of psychopathology, including unipolar and bipolar affective illness, anxiety disorder, and alcoholism, show more ambiguous results. Six of nine studies examining the risk of affective disorders found no significant difference between relatives of patients with schizophrenia or schizoaffective disorder and controls, consistent with the generally accepted dichotomy between psychotic and affective illness. It is important to note, however, that a third of studies did detect excess risk of affective disorders. Five of six studies of risk of anxiety disorders in relatives found no significant differences. Four of five studies of alcoholism found no significant increase in risk. A twin study that explored the DSM-III definition of schizophrenia found evidence of an increased degree of genetic determination when concordance was broadened to include categories such as schizophreniform and atypical psychosis. However when co-twins with a broader range of conditions, including major depression, were included as "affected," the evidence of a genetic effect, as reflected in the monozygotic to dizygotic concordance ratio, fell markedly (Farmer et al. 1987).

Answers to the question of diagnostic breadth are particularly important for molecular genetic investigation of schizophrenia, since they specify who is considered affected. Misclassification of affected individuals causes great loss in power to detect genetic effects. As is clear from the summary above, the boundaries of psychiatric illnesses are unclear, and consequently, we do not know exactly where to set definitions of illness for classifying individuals. There is obviously a great difference between calling a pair of siblings affected if both are diagnosed with schizophrenia and calling the same pair affected if one is diagnosed with schizophrenia and the other with a personality disorder, or one with schizophrenia and the other with alcoholism. Though the field as a whole concurs that we do not know where to set the boundary, the approximation we choose in the meantime is the source of considerable controversy. It has become reasonably common to perform several analyses of data with a number of different definitions of illness. This has the benefits of allowing different genes to influence different ranges of pathology and of making no assumptions about the range of pathology to which any gene predisposes a person.

Methods: Where and How Will Such Genes Be Found?

Linkage and association are two fundamentally different genetic effects with quite different strategies for their detection. Both are widely used in the search for schizophrenia susceptibility genes. The major difference between these two approaches is that association studies are generally focused on candidate genes (or more recently regions), whereas linkage studies make no assumption about specific genes involved in etiology. Because of their fundamental differences, the two approaches have generally been considered separately. A recent and very important shift in the field is that, increasingly, association studies have tended to follow linkage evidence. The sequential application of these two approaches has produced the most exciting current results, including identification of a small but growing number of specific genes, which we focus on here, for which multiple groups have found support. These topics should therefore be treated as related rather than separate.

Linkage Analysis

Classical single-gene, or Mendelian, genetic illnesses are caused by a single faulty gene, located at a single place on a chromosome. Because these illnesses are rare, the rare risk allele must *segregate* (or pass) from parents with a family history into affected offspring or arise as an even rarer de novo mutation. By following the segregation of marker alleles from the affected lineage into offspring, chromosome regions from which affected offspring inherit one marker allele and unaffected offspring the other can be identified. This phenomenon of chromosomal regions segregating with a trait in multiple families is termed *linkage*. It is detectable because there is *crossover* (i.e., a physical exchange of material) between the chromosome pairs during *meiosis*, the cell division resulting in the production of eggs or sperm. *Recombination*, the occurrence of chromosomes with new combinations of alleles, is observed genetically and is the result of this crossover (Figure 3–2). It also provides the measure of genetic distance most commonly used, the *centimorgan* (cM), which is equivalent to 1% recombination between two loci. If two genetic loci are on different chromosomes, the probability that they are inherited together will be 0.5. This means that the theoretical maximum genetic distance is 50 cM. This phenomenon of *independent assortment*, as Mendel described it, is also true for two loci far apart on the same chromosome when there is an even chance that they will be separated by crossovers at meiosis. On the other hand, linkage is observed between two loci when they are in such close proximity on the same chromosome that their alleles are separated by crossing over less than half the time. In other words, there is a departure from independent assortment (Figure 3–3), which can be statistically tested for.

Methods

Two different forms of linkage analyses are in common use. *Parametric* analyses require the specification of a genetic model. When these models can be specified accurately, parametric linkage is a powerful approach. However, the difficulties discussed earlier in defining a transmission model and specifying who should be considered affected suggest that it is much less powerful for analysis of schizophrenia. The parametric linkage statistic is the *LOD* (logarithm of the odds) *score*. A LOD score is the logarithm, to the base 10, of the ratio of the likelihood of the observed data given linkage divided by the likelihood of that same data given no linkage. A LOD score of +3 (which corresponds to a genomewide significance level of $P=0.05$ [Morton 1955; see also Lander and Kruglyak 1995]) indicates that the likelihood that the observed families are linked is 1,000 times the likelihood that they are un-

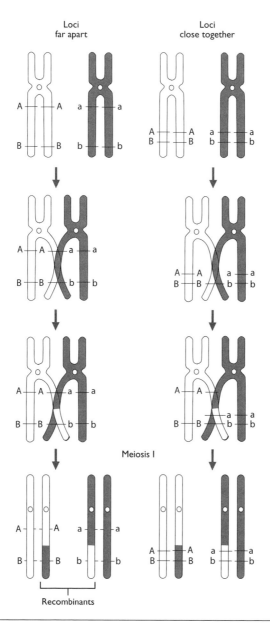

Loci
far apart

Loci
close together

Meiosis I

Recombinants

Figure 3–2. Recombination between homologous chromosomes in meiosis.

The left diagram illustrates two loci that are far apart on the same chromosome. These loci have an even chance that they will be separated by crossovers at meiosis. On the right, the two loci are close together so they are less likely to recombine.

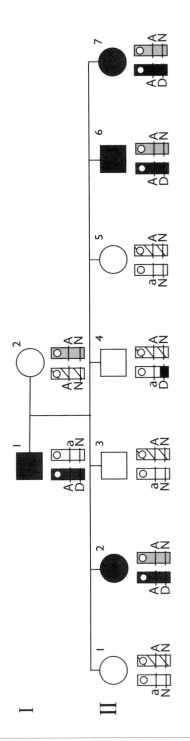

Figure 3–3. Linkage between a disease gene and marker locus close together on the same chromosome.

Allele D is a dominantly inherited disease gene, whereas N is the normal allele at the disease locus. A and a are alternative alleles at a marker locus. Individuals indicated by a solid symbol are affected by disease. Among three of the four affected offspring, the disease gene (D) is inherited with the marker allele A. The three unaffected offspring inherit the normal allele (N) along with the marker allele a. These individuals demonstrate linkage between the two loci. However, individual II-4 is a recombinant because D has been inherited along with a; crossover has occurred between the disease locus and marker locus in the paternal meiosis.

linked (and the likelihood ratio is 10^3, or 1,000:1); a LOD score of −2 (which is generally accepted as significant evidence against linkage) means that the likelihood that the observed families are unlinked is 100 times the likelihood that they are linked (and the likelihood ratio is thus 10^{-2}, or 0.01:1). Because linkage analysis is likelihood-based and likelihood-based tests can be maximized over one or more parameters, a common technique is to vary parameters and use likelihood maximization to choose the best parameter value. Thus, the focus of linkage analysis is often comparison of the relative likelihood of the data under one parameter value compared with another.

Variations of the LOD score that allow for heterogeneity, or that assess only the affected individuals in a sample, have been applied to address some of the problems outlined above, but we will not distinguish between these in the discussion that follows. An alternative approach, widely used in complex traits, is *nonparametric* linkage analysis. All classes of relatives have predefined probabilities of sharing zero, one, or two alleles at a random marker locus. These nonparametric statistics, which are based on testing for deviations from expected allele-sharing distributions, avoid the problem of specifying a model, which, as we saw above, is very difficult for schizophrenia.

Challenges in Applying Linkage Analysis to Schizophrenia

Linkage has proven to be a method of immense power for Mendelian disorders in the study of which a small number of families can usually unambiguously produce strong evidence for linkage to a small chromosomal region. Despite years of work, such a result has not emerged for schizophrenia (in common with many complex traits) because, as outlined in Table 3–1, schizophrenia differs from Mendelian disorders in at least five critical ways, all of which make successful linkage studies much more difficult.

1. *Schizophrenia does not have full penetrance.* Most Mendelian disorders have full penetrance. If you inherit a disease mutation and live through the period of risk, you will always suffer from the disorder. As discussed above, the pattern of illness in families (risk of schizophrenia of about 9%–17% in first-degree relatives

Table 3–1. Comparison of classical Mendelian disorders and schizophrenia

Characteristics	Mendelian disorders	Schizophrenia
Penetrance[a]	Usually complete[b]	Incomplete[c]
Phenocopies	Usually absent	Present
Diagnostic boundaries	Clear	Uncertain
Locus heterogeneity within families	Never	Uncertain, but likely
Locus heterogeneity across families	Variable, but often absent	Uncertain, but likely

[a]The probability of illness given the disease-predisposing genotype.
[b]MZ concordance = ~100%.
[c]MZ concordance = 30%–70%.

of schizophrenic probands and MZ twin concordance about 50%) is inconsistent with the action of a highly penetrant SML. Unlike many other familial illnesses (e.g., Alzheimer's disease and breast cancer), for which a well-recognized series of pedigrees exists in which the disorder segregates in a Mendelian manner, there are no pedigrees in which schizophrenia is transmitted as a classical Mendelian disorder. Finally, the offspring of unaffected MZ co-twins have an elevated risk of illness, suggesting that cases of schizophrenia cannot be simply divided into genetic and *sporadic* (or nongenetic) forms. These results all suggest that, in aggregate, genes involved in the etiology of schizophrenia have reduced penetrance: people can carry risk alleles for schizophrenia and not manifest the illness. For this reason, we call these *liability, susceptibility,* or *predisposing alleles.*

2. *Manifestation of symptoms like those of schizophrenia can result from numerous causes.* For most Mendelian conditions, the manifestation of typical symptoms of the disease is due to the disease mutation. For schizophrenia, this is not true, as schizophrenia-like symptoms can be produced by drugs of abuse and more rarely by metabolic or neurological conditions. Such cases are called *phenocopies.*

3. *Development of schizophrenia is not independent of the environment.* In nearly all Mendelian disorders, disease development is independent of the environment. In schizophrenia, however, environmental factors are critical in accounting for observed patterns of risk. Several environmental risk factors, including obstetric complications and intrauterine influenza infections, have been suggested to increase risk of illness, but large studies of these factors have generally not provided conclusive support.

4. *Schizophrenia, unlike most Mendelian disorders, does not have clearly delineated diagnostic boundaries.* In most Mendelian disorders, individuals are either affected or not and there is a clear distinction between those states. Diagnostic boundaries are less clearly delineated for psychiatric illness and are the subject of continued debate. As noted earlier, we are uncertain of the correct phenotypic boundaries to use for schizophrenia in linkage and association studies.

5. *Susceptibility to develop schizophrenia is not determined by a single gene.* The mutations that cause most Mendelian disorders are sufficiently rare that for all practical purposes, the same disease gene will be responsible for all the cases of illness in a pedigree. Schizophrenia is much more common, and it is plausible, although unproven, that in many high-density families two or more genes are contributing to disease susceptibility. Across families, the pattern with Mendelian disorders is variable. In most disorders, mutations at a single gene are responsible for all known cases of illness (e.g., Huntington's disease, cystic fibrosis). However, for some Mendelian syndromes (e.g., limb-girdle muscular dystrophy and retinitis pigmentosa), a number of distinct genes, usually on different chromosomes, have been found in different subsets of families. Critically, within an individual family the same gene and mutation are responsible for all cases of disease. Given that schizophrenia is not a disease, but rather a broad behavioral syndrome, and given the great complexity of the human brain, it is plausible that mutations in many different genes might result in this condition. This particular issue has a number of ramifications, which merit discussion.

Epidemiological data on schizophrenia suggest that the population frequencies of liability variants are likely to be orders of magnitude greater than the frequency of even the most common single-gene mutations (as with cystic fibrosis, which has a carrier frequency of 2.5%). The implication is that even within families, variants in both shared and distinct genes may predispose different affected family members to illness. Current models hypothesize that variants in many genes can increase liability to schizophrenia (a *polygenic* model of total population risk) and that a few of these genes predispose an individual to schizophrenia (an *oligogenic* model of individual risk). Our current approaches treat loci individually, but the risk associated with an individual gene is likely to be small and may be dependent on the genotypes at other genes (an *epistatic* model of risk). The evidence supporting both polygenic and epistatic models of risk suggests that an additional problem is *stochastic sampling variation*—the random variation of predisposing genes represented in family or case-control samples. This variation (along with concerns about the power of small samples) is widely believed to be responsible for much of the difficulty in replicating linkage results.

In summary, the tight one-to-one relationship that exists between disease mutation and phenotype that is characteristic of Mendelian genetic disorders does not apply to schizophrenia. Locus heterogeneity both within and between families is likely to further complicate this picture. These problems all mean that the *signal-to-noise ratio* for linkage studies will be much greater for schizophrenia. As is true in any experimental design, the lower the signal-to-noise ratio, the larger the sample size that is required to reliably detect an effect. This principle is particularly applicable to linkage studies of complex diseases like schizophrenia. As has been demonstrated by a range of formal power analyses, much larger sample sizes are likely to be required to detect linkage reliably for schizophrenia than were needed for the genetically simple Mendelian disorders. All of these issues should be borne in mind when assessing the evidence for specific chromosomal locations that follows.

Association Studies

Association studies examine whether individuals affected by a disease more frequently have a particular allele at some candidate gene than do individuals who are not affected by the disease. This association can occur for two reasons: either the allele being studied directly influences risk for the disorder, or, more commonly, the allele is in *linkage disequilibrium* with the disease-predisposing mutation. Linkage disequilibrium means that specific alleles at two nearby loci tend to occur together in an entire population. *Linkage*—the co-segregation of a chromosome region and a disease observed in families—occurs at scales of tens of millions of base pairs, whereas *association* (and linkage disequilibrium) is seen at scales of tens of thousands of base pairs. Linkage disequilibrium is a reflection of an evolutionary history in which, because of these very small distances, recombination occurs very rarely between the two loci. Linkage disequilibrium occurs because a new variant (i.e., polymorphic marker or mutation) always arises on a specific background chromosome and will, until separated by recombination, only exist in conjunction with the other alleles present on that background.

In addition, association can occur for spurious reasons unrelated to disease etiology, such as *population stratification,* in which the cases and controls come from different population groups or subgroups, and observed genotypic differences are due to this population difference rather than to true association between marker and phenotype.

Methods

Association approaches have two important advantages when compared with linkage. First, individual patients can be studied rather than families. Second, under many circumstances, a sample of equal size has considerably more power to detect association than to detect linkage to a gene of modest effect. However, association approaches have two potential disadvantages as well. First, association studies can examine only much smaller regions of the genome than linkage. Practically, this means that association studies must be used for the assessment of candidate genes or regions only. Affordable methods for providing genomewide association data are only now becoming widely available. Second, obtaining proper controls for association studies can be difficult and can lead to false positives (through population stratification). This particular issue, although real, appears less significant than once thought, as the conditions necessary to produce false positive findings probably occur only rarely in human populations.

A number of analytical developments have improved association studies. *Transmission disequilibrium testing* (TDT) (Spielman and Ewens 1996) assesses whether certain alleles or *haplotypes* (i.e., the combination of alleles on one of the pair of chromosomes) are transmitted to affected individuals more often than expected by chance. *Pedigree disequilibrium testing* (PDT) (Martin et al. 2000) uses both the transmission information and the information on discordant siblings. Both these approaches have furthered the pursuit of association studies in family samples that were originally collected for linkage studies. The problems of random sampling variation and heterogeneity (among others) all suggest that the best place to follow up a linkage finding is in the family sample that produced it.

Challenges in Applying Association Studies to Schizophrenia

Association studies in schizophrenia (and other psychiatric disorders) have tended to focus on a limited set of "usual suspect" genes, generally those coding for receptors, transporters, and synthetic or degradatory enzymes in neurotransmitter pathways. Results from these studies have generally been neither particularly exciting nor robust, and few replicated findings have emerged to date. Although association studies remain a major interest in attempting to clarify the nature of the genetic liability to schizophrenia, it is probably fair to conclude that a powerful, widely replicated finding has yet to emerge from this technique alone.

Results: Where Is the Evidence Strongest for Schizophrenia Susceptibility Genes?

Twenty-five complete or nearly complete genome scans for schizophrenia (in which about 400 individual genetic markers are genotyped at regular intervals over the entire human genome) have now been published, and none has revealed evidence for a gene of major effect for schizophrenia—results consistent with the evidence reviewed in the previous section. A smaller number of genome scans examining specific clinical features of the illness (e.g., neuropsychological deficits; age at onset; and positive, negative, and disorganized symptoms) have been published. Finally, two meta-analyses of genome scan data using different statistical approaches and six meta-analyses of specific chromosomal regions have been published.

A very brief review of genetic marker types and their designations provides the context for the discussion that follows. Most of the results summarized below come from studies of a particular kind of DNA polymorphism, the *tandem repeat*. Tandem repeats are variable numbers of a repeating unit of nucleotides. Tandem repeat units exist in all sizes, from mononucleotides (rarely used due to the difficulty of accurate genotyping) through dinucleotides (the most common and most commonly used), tri-, tetra-, and pentanucleotides. The frequency of polymorphisms of various unit sizes in the genome is generally inversely correlated with the length of the tandem repeat unit. They are referred to variously as *microsatellites, short tandem repeats, simple sequence repeats*, or *AC repeats* (after the most common dinucleotide repeat sequence). The alleles of these markers are different segment lengths as a result of different numbers of the tandemly repeated unit. This marker type is very common and tends to be extremely polymorphic (i.e., to have many alleles) and therefore to have high *heterozygosity* (i.e., the proportion of individuals who have two different alleles at the marker locus). As a result of the high heterozygosity, it also tends to be extremely *informative,* by which we mean that the probability that the allele transmitted to a given offspring from a given parent can be unambiguously determined. Most linkage studies use microsatellite markers. Nomenclature for markers of this type are "D numbers" that identify the chromosome on which the marker locus maps and the historical order in which the marker was identified. Thus, the 278th microsatellite identified on chromosome 22 (to be discussed shortly) will have D number D22S278.

In contrast, single-nucleotide polymorphisms (SNPs) are genetic variations at a single base and have only two alleles and have lower heterozygosity and lower information content. Association and linkage disequilibrium studies tend, in general, to use SNPs as the marker of choice; whereas large numbers of alleles (and therefore high information content) are useful for linkage, lower allele numbers and lower information content are more appropriate for association studies. Nomenclature for these markers varies, but here we use the "common allele–position–rare allele" convention. A variant with A as the more frequent allele and G as the rarer allele at base 18 of a hypothetical gene would be named A18G. The first base of the methionine *start codon* (the first unit of a gene incorporated in the protein) is always given the number 1. Bases in the upstream region before the start codon are given negative numbers. Where SNPs occur in coding sequence and alter amino acid sequence, they will often be based on the amino acid change and position rather than the nucleotide change and position (Ser311Cys polymorphism in the D_2 receptor gene vs. the T102C polymorphism in the serotonin$_{2A}$ [5-HT$_{2A}$] receptor gene). Finally, we follow standard nomenclature for distinguishing between genes and their protein products. Proteins are designated with either the full name (e.g., catechol-*O*-methyltransferase) or the abbreviation (COMT); protein symbols are always in upper case, ordinary font. Where a protein has more than one name in current use in the literature (e.g., the approved nomenclature "dystrobrevin binding protein 1" and the widely used "dysbindin"), both will be given. Gene symbols are often the same as protein abbreviations but are always given in upper case italics (*COMT*). We will also try to make it clear in the text when we are discussing the gene versus the protein.

Within the last several years, the first tentative evidence for replicated linkage for schizophrenia susceptibility genes has emerged. To date, eight regions appear most promising (in the order they were identified): 22q12-q13, 8p22-p21, 6p24-p22, 13q14-q32, 5q22-q31, 10p15-p11, 6q21-q22, and 15q13-q14. We must note that the interpretation of these results is controversial, particularly as the definition of replication for linkage to a complex trait remains uncertain (Baron 1996; Kendler et al. 1996). In the interest of brevity, studies that do not find evidence for linkage in these selected regions have been omitted, but it is important to bear this selective bias in mind when considering the data that follow. Many samples do not provide supportive evidence for these regions. We have additionally omitted discussion of a number of other less well supported regions; more detailed information about these and other putative linkage regions can be found elsewhere (Riley and McGuffin 2000).

Chromosome 22q Linkage Studies

Evidence for Linkage

Initial evidence for linkage to chromosome 22q came from three markers spanning ~23 cM in the 22q13.1 region in the Maryland family sample (Pulver et al. 1994b). A collaborative replication study in a total of 217 multiplex pedigrees with groups from Virginia, Great Britain, and France followed but did not confirm the linkage in the new samples (Pulver et al. 1994a).

From a number of attempted replications, two samples were positive: pedigrees from Utah (Coon et al. 1994) and from England and Wales (Polymeropoulos et al. 1994). After the size of the Maryland family sample was increased, the most significant marker in their genome scan was the same dinucleotide repeat polymorphism, D22S278, as that showing maximum evidence for linkage in the British and Welsh families. Eleven groups contributed data for this marker to the first collaborative schizophrenia linkage study. Excess sharing of alleles was found in these 620 affected sib pairs ($P=0.006$), particularly in 296 pairs with data available from both parents ($P=0.001$). It is important to note, however, that the authors calculated that this locus is likely to account for no more than 2% of total variance in liability (Gill et al. 1996). The role of this region in liability to schizophrenia remains unclear, although the positive findings seem unlikely to have occurred by chance.

Additional interest in this region of 22q came from a known chromosomal rearrangement. The co-segregation of chromosomal anomalies or rearrangements with phenotypes resembling a particular disease has provided useful clues to the locations of the gene(s) involved, most notably in the positional cloning of the dystrophin gene (*DMD*). Velocardiofacial syndrome (VCFS) is caused by deletions at 22q11, a locus near the region of risk for schizophrenia identified by linkage analysis. Historically, about 10% of VCFS patients were thought to present with a psychotic phenotype, but more recent studies suggest much higher rates of 25%–29% (Murphy et al. 1999; Pulver et al. 1994c). Conversely, preliminary results suggest that about 2% of adult-onset and 6% of childhood-onset schizophrenia patients have microdeletions in this region, in excess of the estimated general population frequency of such deletions (0.025%) (Karayiorgou et al. 1995). Although statistically significant, this excess of deletions is probably not enough to explain significant *population attributable risk* (PAR), but variation in genes in this region in individuals without a deletion may contribute to liability.

Chromosome 22q Candidate Genes: COMT

The VCFS critical region contains the gene for catechol-*O*-methyltransferase (*COMT*), located at 22q11, which is involved in the synthesis and degradation of catecholamines and is genetically and functionally polymorphic, with a variable amino acid, Val158Met. Val and Met alleles are of almost identical frequency. Most studies of *COMT* have tested for association with the low activity (Met) allele (with mixed results). One report suggested that the high-activity (Val) allele, through increased catabolism of dopamine in the prefrontal cortex, may slightly increase the risk of schizophrenia and may explain some of the observed differences in cognitive performance and prefrontal cortical functioning between cases and control subjects (Egan et al. 2001).

Another study examined *COMT* in a homogeneous population of Ashkenazi Jewish individuals from Israel and used the largest case-control sample for schizophrenia yet reported (Shifman et al. 2002). Three of these SNPs genotyped in *COMT* showed significant association with schizophrenia in ~720 cases and 2,000–4,000 controls. In agreement with Egan et al.'s (2001) study discussed above, an association was found with the homozygous high-activity genotype (Val/Val) and with the two other SNPs tested. Interestingly, differences between men and women for allele and genotype frequencies, strength of association, and PAR were seen at all three loci individually and in haplotype analyses. Overall, the study found that the PAR for *COMT* in females was 32.2%, while that in males was 13.5%. Although the PAR estimates need to be interpreted with caution because of the evidence for an epistatic model of risk discussed earlier, they suggest that 32.2% of female patients and 13.5% of male patients would not have been affected if liability variants in this gene had not been present in the population. No such observation of a differential effect of a gene in males and females had previously been reported.

Chromosome 8p22-p21 Linkage Studies

Evidence for Linkage

The Maryland family sample also gave the first evidence of linkage to chromosome 8p22-p21 (Pulver et al. 1995). A multicenter collaborative linkage study supported this putative locus with excess allele sharing at D8S261 (Levinson et al. 1996). Data from pedigrees from numerous different ethnic backgrounds all support a locus on 8p. These replication results are spread across about 15 Mb of sequence. One of the key points to note is that although numerous samples support a locus on this chromosome, comparison between individual studies is consistent with the possibility of multiple genes in the region.

Chromosome 8p22-p21 Candidate Genes: NRG1

Following linkage evidence to chromosome 8p in Icelandic families, fine mapping with 50 markers across a 30-cM interval identified two risk haplotypes spanning a region of ~1 Mb within the gene for neuregulin 1 (*NRG1*) (Stefansson et al. 2002). Case-control samples from Scotland (Stefansson et al. 2003) and Ireland (Corvin et al. 2004) have provided additional support for this locus and for haplotypes identical or closely related to those identified in the Icelandic cases. Studies in other populations have provided support for this association (Bakker et al. 2004; Li et al. 2004; Tang et al. 2004; Williams et al. 2003; Yang et al. 2003; Zhao et al. 2004), though not with the specific haplotypes seen in the

Icelandic, Scottish, and Irish samples. Neuregulin is expressed in CNS synapses and appears to have a role in the expression and activation of neurotransmitter (including glutamate) receptors.

Chromosome 6p24-p22 Linkage Studies

Evidence for Linkage

The first evidence for linkage of schizophrenia to the 6p region came from studies of Irish families with a high density of disease (Straub et al. 1995). In data based on 16 markers, evidence for linkage was modest under a narrow diagnostic model but increased substantially as the diagnostic definition broadened to include spectrum disorders. Evidence for linkage fell when the definition was broadened further to include nonspectrum disorders. The relationship between diagnostic breadth and evidence for linkage in this sample is illustrated in Figure 3–4.

To date, eight independent reports of analyses of this region of 6p have been published. Studies of German and mixed German and Israeli pedigrees supported linkage to 6p24-p22 (Moises et al. 1995; Schwab et al. 1995). Analysis of a family sample from Quebec found supportive evidence for a schizophrenia susceptibility locus in some but not all families (Maziade et al. 1997). A large, multigeneration family from Sweden supported this linkage in a single branch of the family; a haplotype of markers within the putative linked segment was found to segregate with schizophrenia (Lindholm et al. 1999). A large, multicenter collaboration detected significant excess allele sharing in this region (Levinson et al. 1996).

Chromosome 6p24-p22 Candidate Genes: DTNBP1

Follow-up work in the Irish family set demonstrated a positive association in the dystrobrevin binding protein 1, or dysbindin, gene (*DTNBP1*) (Straub et al. 2002). Subsequent reanalysis of the association data revealed a risk haplotype of SNP markers in this gene (van den Oord et al. 2003). Replication studies have been generally supportive of these findings (Funke et al. 2004; Kirov et al. 2004; Kendler 2004; Kohn et al. 2004; Schwab et al. 2003; Tang et al. 2003; Van Den Bogaert et al. 2003; Williams et al. 2004a).

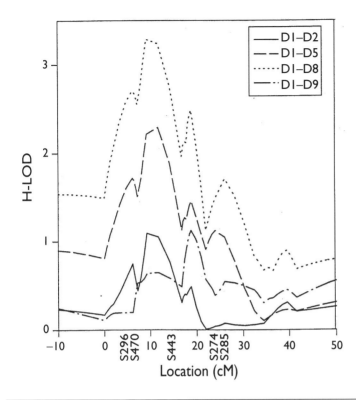

Figure 3–4. Relationship between diagnostic breadth and evidence for linkage on chromosome 6p in the Irish High Density Family Sample.

The function of dystrobrevin binding protein 1 is unknown, and the protein must currently be considered in relation to the proteins it is known to interact with. It was first identified as a binding partner of both a- and b-dystrobrevins (Benson et al. 2001), which are binding partners of dystrophin, a large, membrane-associated protein expressed at its highest levels in muscle and brain and mutated in Duchenne and Becker muscular dystrophy (Ray et al. 1985). In muscle, dystrophin is associated with the dystrophin-associated protein complex (DPC), which spans the membrane and links the cytoskeleton and the extracellular matrix. Dystrophin is central to the formation of the DPC, and in addition to mechanical function, the DPC is thought to be involved in intracellular signaling. However, several lines of evidence suggest that the mechanisms of action for these molecules may be different in neuronal and muscle tissue and may be different in different regions of the brain. Current evidence suggests that the expression of *DTNBP1* is reduced in certain brain regions of patients with schizophrenia at both the RNA (Weickert et al. 2004) and protein (Talbot et al. 2004) levels.

Chromosome 13q14-q32 Linkage Studies

Evidence for Linkage

Data from a mixed sample of U.K. and Japanese families initially suggested linkage of schizophrenia to chromosome 13q14.1-q32 (Lin et al. 1995), of interest as the region contains the 5-HT$_{2A}$ receptor gene. Preliminary data from the Maryland and U.K./Icelandic samples gave some initial support for this linkage (Antonarakis et al. 1996; Kalsi et al. 1996). An attempt by the original group to replicate in an independent sample of Taiwanese and U.K. families supported the finding only in the European families (Lin et al. 1997). Further analyses of the European sample using slightly different methods yielded positive data at two markers located at 13q32, but they were separated by a region where the values of the statistics dropped almost to zero.

Genome scan data from a mixed U.K./U.S. sample gave positive evidence of linkage, but extremely distant from other findings in the region (Shaw et al. 1998). The Maryland family sample gave modest evidence for linkage under a recessive model; nonparametric analysis of the same data was highly significant. Marker data in narrowly defined Canadian pedigrees gave fairly strong evidence for linkage (Brzustowicz et al. 1999). The results from chromosome 13 are particularly difficult to interpret because of the very large distances between positive markers. Unlike chromosome 6, where 2 distinct regions have been detected in different samples, there has been little agreement about the site of greatest evidence on 13q. Overall, the combined linkage reports are spread over a region of ~60 Mb, containing ~120 known or putative genes. However, although locations are much less certain on chromosome 13q than in other linkage regions, this chromosome has produced some of the most significant linkage evidence seen in the studies of schizophrenia.

Chromosome 13q14-q32 Candidate Genes: G72 and DAAO

An elegant study examined markers in the distal 5 Mb of this broad linkage region, site of one of the most significant findings on chromosome 13 (Chumakov et al. 2002). Nearly 200 SNPs were tested across the region, and the testing identified two regions of association. In one of these regions, two genes, *G72* and *G30*, were investigated. Of note, the exons of these genes could not be predicted by any computational method tested, suggesting that they are highly novel in their sequence and organization. Both genes show alternative transcripts in brain and other tissues. Association studies of SNPs within *G72* have not yet provided a clear pattern. One of these is nonsynonymous and is significant alone. The nature of the amino acid change (lysine to arginine) is conservative but has major consequences in some proteins. However, the overall pattern of results is probably most consistent with the existence of further unidentified predisposing variants in this gene.

D-Amino acid oxidase (DAAO) was identified as a binding partner of, and appears to be activated by, the protein product of *G72*. *DAAO*, on chromosome 12q24, was screened for association evidence, and four SNPs tested were significantly associated. Results of this kind (showing association in two interacting genes in the same sample) are rare, so this study had a unique opportunity to test for an epistatic genetic interaction. Evidence for epistasis was observed for one pair of *DAAO* and *G72* genotypes, supporting a potential interaction between them in risk for schizophrenia. Replication studies have generally provided confirmation of a role for *G72* (Addington et al. 2004; Korostishevsky et al. 2004; Schumacher et al. 2004; Wang et al. 2004).

Chromosome 5q22-q31 Linkage Studies

Evidence for Linkage

The first widely noted positive evidence for linkage in schizophrenia, and the first study to use DNA polymorphisms, was reported by Sherrington et al. in 1988. Following up on the report of an association of schizophrenia with a partial trisomy of chromosome 5q, they examined the proximal region of the trisomy, including the 5q11.2 breakpoint, with two restriction-length polymorphisms (RFLPs) in seven U.K. and Icelandic families. The strong evidence they reported for linkage in this region could not, however, be replicated by many other groups nor by the original investigators themselves.

Two groups have found suggestive evidence of linkage on chromosome 5q22-q31 in a region distinct from that in earlier studies. Data from the Irish sample were positive under a narrow diagnostic model. Analyses with a broader disease definition resulted in substantial reduction in the statistics. Results were positive (though of variable magnitude) across the entire set of 14 markers spanning 45 cM of this region (Straub et al. 1997).

Markers in the same region gave positive results in families from Germany and, subsequently, in families from Germany and Israel (including four from the first sample) at markers 2 cM apart. Excess allele sharing was observed over a region of 8 cM. A single case of an individual with mental retardation and schizophrenia who had a deletion of this chromosome region has also been reported (Schwab et al. 1997).

Chromosome 10p15-p11 Linkage Studies

Genome screen data from U.S. families of European descent produced the most suggestive finding on chromosome 10p15-q21 (Faraone et al. 1998). Data from the Irish and German and Israeli families provided further evidence for a 10p susceptibility locus (Schwab et al. 1998; Straub et al. 1998). Excess allele sharing was seen over a number of markers in the latter sample. The results from 5q and 10p were unusual because of the close agreement (within 5 cM) in samples using different diagnostic and analytical approaches.

Chromosome 6q21-q22 Linkage Studies

A sample of 53 U.S. families provided initial evidence for a susceptibility locus on chromosome 6q21-q22.3 (Cao et al. 1997). This study is unique in that a second independent sample of families held by the same researchers was used to replicate the finding internally and supported the results from the first sample. A further replication study by the same group found positive but less significant maxima in a third independent sample (Martinez et al. 1999). When the data from both replication samples were combined, an interval of ~8 Mb gave the strongest results under both parametric and nonparametric approaches, with a LOD of 3.82 and highly significant excess allele sharing.

Data from the African American pedigrees in the NIMH/Millenium Schizophrenia Genome Screen provided support for these findings (Kaufmann et al. 1998). The markers positive in this latter sample flank the 8 Mb region of interest described above. A collaborative study of these last four regions gave highly significant evidence for a schizophrenia susceptibility locus on 6q21-q22 and modest support across a much larger region of chromosome 10p, but did not support a locus on 5q or 13q (Levinson et al. 2000).

The group that provided initial evidence for a susceptibility locus on chromosome 6q21-q22.3 followed up their linkage findings with linkage dysequilibrium studies in the same samples and identified association in the trace amine receptor 4 gene (*TRAR4*) located at 6q23.2 (Duan et al. 2004). Although at the time of writing this finding remains to be replicated by other groups, we have included it because it represents continuous work from linkage to candidate gene identification and testing by the same group in the same samples. As we have seen, the results from such work have tended to be robust, in contrast to those from a number of high-profile candidate genes identified through other means (Emamian et al. 2004; Gerber et al. 2003; Liu et al. 2002), which have been difficult to replicate.

Chromosome 15q13-q14 Linkage Studies

The first evidence for a possible chromosome 15 schizophrenia susceptibility locus was the report of linkage of an evoked potential abnormality common in patients with schizophrenia and relatively rare in control subjects to chromosome 15q13-q14 (Freedman et al. 1997). The abnormality is thought to reflect a sensory gating deficit (i.e., a decreased capacity to filter out repetitive stimuli), and it segregates as a single gene trait in families. Linkage evidence was strongest for a marker in intron 2 of the α7 nicotinic cholinergic receptor subunit gene (*CHRNA7*), which gave a highly significant LOD score when tested against the sensory gating phenotype, and a positive but nonsignificant LOD when tested against schizophrenia. In addition to the positional evidence, this gene is an attractive candidate because of the high incidence of smoking in patients with schizophrenia and because both nicotine and clozapine ameliorate the sensory gating deficit.

Data from South African Bantu families in a dense marker set around *CHRNA7* gave positive nonparametric evidence across the entire map. Analysis of marker haplotypes in the Bantu families gave significant evidence for overtransmission of one marker haplotype to affected individuals, consistent with a susceptibility allele existing on this haplotype (Riley et al. 2000). Analyses by the original group in an independent sample detected highly significant excess allele sharing at D15S1360 (Leonard et al. 1998).

Four subsequent studies found additional supportive evidence for a susceptibility locus in this region in Taiwanese families (Liu et al. 2001), a Veterans Affairs Cooperative sample (Tsuang et al. 2001), Azorean families (Xu et al. 2001), and another sample of U.S. families (Gejman et al. 2001). The last result is some distance away from the others, which are tightly clustered around *CHRNA7*. Screening of the *CHRNA7* promoter region for polymorphisms has shown that the identified variants all reduce expression of *CHRNA7* and that the variants are significantly more common in cases than in controls (Gault et al. 1999). Sensory gating was significantly poorer in those controls with a promoter variant than in the controls without.

Chromosomes 9q34.3, 4q24-q32, 18, and 1q32-q41

Four additional chromosome regions deserve brief mention, although the evidence for their involvement in schizophrenia is less well replicated and less certain. Two studies have found positive evidence on chromosome 9q34.3 very close to the q-telomere. This region contains two genes of potential interest, the dopamine β-hydroxylase gene (*DBH*) and the gene for a central subunit of the NMDA receptor (*NR1*). The first of these was tested directly in one sample, and no positive evidence was obtained. However, both neurochemical and transgenic mouse studies support a possible role for *NR1* in liability to schizophrenia.

In one sample, a cluster of three markers on 4q24-q32 gave some evidence for involvement in liability to schizophrenia. This region has been a focus of attention in studies of bipolar disorder. Some evidence in support of this region was observed in Irish, U.S. and Australian, and Finnish family samples.

Interest in chromosome 18 began with several reports of the co-occurrence of psychiatric disorders and chromosomal anomalies, and linkage evidence between this chromosome and bipolar disorder has also been reported. Two replication attempts in schizophrenia samples following the putative bipolar linkage were negative, but several positive results have been reported in markers and candidate genes in the German/Israeli sample with and without the inclusion of affective disorder families and in data from Welsh families.

Interest in chromosome 1 in schizophrenia began with reports of a balanced 1:11 translocation segregating with serious mental illness in a large pedigree from Scotland. The chromosome 1 breakpoint lies at 1q42.1, and two groups reported suggestive linkage findings in this region—in a population isolate from Finland (Hovatta et al. 1999) and in the Maryland sample. Ongoing work in the Scottish pedigree has now identified three genes disrupted by the breakpoint (and of potential interest in psychotic illness more generally) in this region (Millar et al. 2000). Genome scans of families from Finland and Canada have also provided evidence for a chromosome 1 locus, although the chromosomal position varies between these studies and thus interpretation is difficult. The last of these (Brzustowicz et al. 2000) provided very strong LOD scores, but their findings were not replicated by a large collaborative study (Levinson et al. 2002).

Microarray studies of postmortem schizophrenic brain suggested that *RGS4*, a regulator of G-protein signaling, altered expression in schizophrenia (Mirnics et al. 2001). *RGS4* maps to the chromosome 1 linkage region, and in a subsequent study in mixed U.S. pedigrees and samples from India, the same markers in the same 10-kilobase region were associated in both samples, although different specific marker haplotypes led to this evidence in the U.S.

pedigrees compared with the Indian families (Chowdari et al. 2002). Replication studies of the *RGS4* locus have also provided support for the association of *RGS4* with schizophrenia liability (Chen et al. 2004; Morris et al. 2004; Williams et al. 2004b).

Summary of Current Linkage Regions and Candidate Genes

The linkage and association results we review below share at least two of the following three features: 1) they have been replicated in at least two other samples in addition to the one in which they were first reported; 2) they have not been replicated in all studies; and 3) they have been pooled, in a collaborative effort, across many groups and have produced suggestive results. These regions represent a wide range of results: narrow (5q, 10p, 15q) to very broad (8p, 13q) regions of chromosomes; those supported (6p, 6q, 8p) or not (5q, 13q) by replication in collaborative studies; and those with positive evidence in candidate genes (22q, 6p, 8p, 10p, 13q, 15q) and those without (5q, 6q). Currently, all the regions and candidate genes discussed in the foregoing sections are promising, but further assessment of each is needed, both to clarify patterns of linkage or association and to elucidate their contribution to the neurobiology of schizophrenia.

The collected evidence for the current best set of candidate genes for schizophrenia susceptibility displays both similarities and contrasts to the summary of linkage evidence presented above. The reported associations for several of these candidates—*DTNBP1*, *NRG1*, *G72*, and *RGS4*—have been replicated in other samples. Critically, positive replications outnumber negative ones for all these loci. Other candidates, such as *COMT* and *TRAR4*, await the collection of sufficient data before an interpretation of the validity of the original studies can be made.

One particularly exciting shared feature of most of the candidates discussed in this section is that they can be related to potential pathophysiology through dysfunction in glutamatergic neurotransmission, which may be an important systemic element in the etiology of schizophrenia. Although a detailed discussion of this theory is outside the scope of this chapter, recent reviews of the genetic (Harrison and Owen 2003) and neuroscience (Moghaddam 2003) evidence discuss the positions of the gene products of *NRG1, COMT, DAAO, G72,* and *RGS4,* among others, in the biochemical and functional pathways influencing the glutamatergic system. More recent work suggests that *DTNBP1* might influence exocytotic glutamate release: overexpression results in increased extracellular basal glutamate levels, while reduced protein expression, as seen in *small interfering RNA* studies in which translation of mRNA into protein is inhibited, results in reduced presynaptic glutamate release (Numakawa et al. 2004).

Meta-analyses of Genome Screen Data

Meta-analysis of whole genome screen data offers a different kind of insight into the mechanisms of complex trait genetics. Because many samples, and therefore more data, are included, meta-analyses represent a first approximation of a very large, multisample genome screen. Two different statistical approaches for such meta-analyses have been published. One combines the significance levels reported in the original genome screens after correction of each value for the size of the suggested region. Four different statistics are calculated with this approach, the most important of which—the replication multiple scan probability—excludes the most significant study (in order to assess the overall evidence without being biased by the most extreme single result). Results from the first approach were significant for chromosomes 8p, 13q, and 22q (Badner and Gershon 2002). The major limitation of this analysis is that it relied only on published results, an approach that prevents critical standardization across the studies. Additionally, in contrast to the second approach below, no new information about potential regions of interest can be extracted with such an approach.

The second method ranks 30-cM bins of the genome from most positive to least positive for each study, and then sums the ranks for each bin. Significance levels are calculated by simulation. Since this method does not use significance levels but rather uses the actual marker LOD scores supplied by each of the investigative groups specifically for these analyses, it is possible to identify regions of the genome that are of potential interest on the basis of modest positive results occurring in the same region across many studies but that may have been overlooked because of the issues of signal-to-noise ratio and stochastic sampling variation discussed earlier. Results of the second approach, which is methodologically the stronger of the two, supported linkage to chromosomes 6p, 8p, and 10p of the previously identified regions discussed above (Lewis et al. 2003).

However, the strongest evidence for a potential locus was on chromosome 2q, a region suggested by only a few studies and not widely followed up, and on 3p, the site of an early linkage finding in the Maryland sample that could not be replicated in subsequent studies. Finally, significant evidence of linkage was also detected for two regions never previously implicated by an individual study, on chromosomes 11q and 14p. These results are currently being followed up.

Discussion

The field of linkage and association studies of schizophrenia continues to change rapidly and may even have altered considerably by the time this chapter is read. Certainly the most important development in the last several years has been the emergence of a number of replicated findings and the identification of associations within genes in these target regions. Given the vast number of statistical tests that are now performed in most linkage studies (e.g., many markers, several diagnostic models, several genetic models, often several different linkage programs), the true type I (or false positive) error rate emerging from any individual study is nearly impossible to quantify. It remains a major concern that results of quite high apparent statistical significance could occur by chance alone because so many tests are performed.

Therefore, replication is critical. However, there are many reasons why a "true" finding might not be replicated, including genetic variation between populations and differences in statistical power, diagnostic methods, and statistical approaches. Given the evidence of replication across several groups for regions on 22q, 8p, 6p, 13q, 5q, 10p, 6q, 1q, and 15q, it seems increasingly unlikely that all of these regions represent false positives. It is difficult to conceive of an inherent bias that would produce spuriously positive results across multiple groups (especially given the wide differences between studies described above) in the same chromosomal region.

A further important development in the field has been the emergence of results from whole genome scans for other complex disorders, including type 1 (Hashimoto et al. 1994) and type 2 (Busfield et al. 2002; Vionnet et al. 2000; Wiltshire et al. 2001) diabetes mellitus, multiple sclerosis (Coraddu et al. 2001; Sawcer et al. 1996), inflammatory bowel disease (Hugot et al. 2001; Ogura et al. 2001), and asthma (Laitinen et al. 2001). These studies may hold important lessons for our attempts to understand schizophrenia. For insulin-dependent diabetes and multiple sclerosis, a "major" gene appears to exist in the HLA region that has been detected in nearly all studies. However, in other regions, nonreplication across groups is as frequent as replication. This is also the pattern seen in initial studies of asthma. One study of asthma, a genome scan in sib pairs from three different U.S. ethnic groups, showed almost no replication for putative regions of linkage across the three samples. These results suggest that the difficulties in detecting replicable linkages for schizophrenia may not be unique to the psychiatric disorders, but rather may reflect a general pattern of problems associated with linkage studies of complex disorders. When the simple and powerful one-to-one relationship between gene and phenotype that is seen in Mendelian disorders breaks down, detecting genes of modest effect size for complex, moderately heritable diseases is likely to prove a difficult task. However, there appears to be cause for some optimism, as the candidates currently under most intense scrutiny are, in general, apparently being replicated.

We have focused here on the molecular genetic study of schizophrenia, since there is already more material from this area alone than can be accommodated by this chapter. In generalizing to other psychiatric (and other complex) phenotypes, the broad conclusions from the study of schizophrenia seem likely to hold:

1. Such phenotypes are genetically influenced but not genetically determined.

2. A number of genes (which may even vary between individual family members) are likely to be involved.
3. The liability variants in these genes are generally expected to be within the range of normal human variation and to have low risk associated with them individually.
4. Some of the variants may interact with other variants or with environmental risk factors.

The genetic epidemiology of other psychiatric traits does, of course, identify patterns specific to the individual phenotype. Autism, for example, appears to be more strongly genetically mediated (probably by more deleterious though much rarer variants, leading to its much lower population prevalence but higher sibling recurrence risk) and may be the most "genetic" of psychiatric phenotypes. However, these differences are likely to be outweighed by the large number of similarities: difficulties with replication studies (particularly those using linkage) and evidence for the involvement of numerous chromosomal regions or specific genes (from linkage and association studies, respectively) and multiple risk pathways that involve specific subsets of the total number of risk loci.

Conclusion

The evidence is strong that schizophrenia is a familial disorder and that the familial aggregation of schizophrenia is due largely, although probably not entirely, to genetic factors. Whatever the nature of the familial predisposition to developing schizophrenia, it not only "codes" for the classic, deteriorating psychotic disorder but also increases liability to "schizophrenia-like" personality disorders and probably for some other nonschizophrenic nonaffective psychoses. Research using statistical methods has failed over the past two decades to clearly delineate the mode of transmission of schizophrenia, a result that is understandable given its likely complexity.

Advances in molecular and statistical genetics have opened up realistic opportunities to localize on the human genome the specific genes that influence the liability to schizophrenia. Association studies have yet to provide convincing evidence for the role of a range of candidate genes in the etiology of schizophrenia. Genome scan strategies have, however, provided several regions, including chromosomes 5q, 6p, 6q, 8p, 10p, 13q, 15q, and 22q, where a number of groups have found evidence for linkage. While false positive findings cannot be ruled out, it is likely that one or more of these regions do contain one or more susceptibility genes for schizophrenia. This belief is supported by findings of an emerging number of identified positional candidate genes that, in some cases, are now being replicated in independent samples. Given the major focus on this area of multiple research groups worldwide, it is likely that within several years these or other loci might emerge as widely replicated susceptibility genes for schizophrenia. If this occurs, it will represent a true watershed event in the history of schizophrenia research.

While the step of gene identification itself signifies a major advance, it also represents the beginning of several new lines of research, including 1) rational drug design based on knowledge of basic pathophysiology, 2) characterization of genotype-phenotype relationships based on knowledge of specific pathogenic mutations, 3) identification of environmental risk factors that interact with specific genes, and 4) realistic prevention research given our ability to identify high-risk individuals.

References

Addington AM, Gornick M, Sporn AL, et al: Polymorphisms in the 13q33.2 gene G72/G30 are associated with childhood-onset schizophrenia and psychosis not otherwise specified. Biol Psychiatry 55: 976–980, 2004

Antonarakis SE, Blouin JL, Curran M, et al: Linkage and sib-pair analysis reveal a potential schizophrenia susceptibility gene on chromosome 13q32 (abstract). Am J Hum Genet 59:A210, 1996

Badner JA, Gershon ES: Meta-analysis of whole-genome linkage scans of bipolar disorder and schizophrenia. Mol Psychiatry 7:405–411, 2002

Bakker SC, Hoogendoorn ML, Selten JP, et al: Neuregulin 1: genetic support for schizophrenia subtypes. Mol Psychiatry 9:1061–1063, 2004

Baron M: Linkage results in schizophrenia. Am J Med Genet 67:121–123, 1996

Benson MA, Newey SE, Martin-Rendon E, et al: Dysbindin, a novel coiled-coil–containing protein that interacts with the dystrobrevins in muscle and brain. J Biol Chem 276:24232–24241, 2001

Brzustowicz LM, Honer WG, Chow EWC, et al: Linkage of familial schizophrenia to chromosome 13q32. Am J Hum Genet 65:1096–1103, 1999

Brzustowicz LM, Hodgkinson KA, Chow EWC, et al: Location of a major susceptibility locus for familial schizophrenia on chromosome 1q21–q22. Science 288:678–682, 2000

Busfield F, Duffy DL, Kesting JB, et al: A genomewide search for type 2 diabetes-susceptibility genes in indigenous Australians. Am J Hum Genet 70:349–357, 2002

Cao Q, Martinez M, Zhang J, et al: Suggestive evidence for a schizophrenia susceptibility locus on chromosome 6q and a confirmation in an independent series of pedigrees. Genomics 43:1–8, 1997

Cardno AG, Gottesman II: Twin studies of schizophrenia: from bow-and-arrow concordances to Star Wars Mx and functional genomics. Am J Med Genet 97:12–17, 2000

Cardno AG, Marshall EJ, Coid B, et al: Heritability estimates for psychotic disorders: the Maudsley twin psychosis series. Arch Gen Psychiatry 56:162–168, 1999

Caspi A, McClay J, Moffitt TE, et al: Role of genotype in the cycle of violence in maltreated children. Science 297:851–854, 2002

Caspi A, Sugden K, Moffitt TE, et al: Influence of life stress on depression: moderation by a polymorphism in the 5-HTT gene. Science 301:386–389, 2003

Chen X, Dunham C, Kendler S, et al: Regulator of G-protein signaling 4 (RGS4) gene is associated with schizophrenia in Irish high density families. Am J Med Genet 129B:23–26, 2004

Chowdari KV, Mirnics K, Semwal P, et al: Association and linkage analyses of RGS4 polymorphisms in schizophrenia. Hum Mol Genet 11:1373–1380, 2002

Chumakov I, Blumenfeld M, Guerassimenko O, et al: Genetic and physiological data implicating the new human gene G72 and the gene for D-amino acid oxidase in schizophrenia. Proc Natl Acad Sci USA 99:13675–13680, 2002

Coon H, Holik J, Hoff M, et al: Analysis of chromosome 22 markers in nine schizophrenia pedigrees. Am J Med Genet 54:72–79, 1994

Coraddu F, Sawcer S, D'Alfonso S, et al: A genome screen for multiple sclerosis in Sardinian multiplex families. Eur J Hum Genet 9:621–626, 2001

Corvin AP, Morris DW, McGhee K, et al: Confirmation and refinement of an 'at-risk' haplotype for schizophrenia suggests the EST cluster, Hs.97362, as a potential susceptibility gene at the neuregulin-1 locus. Mol Psychiatry 9:208–213, 2004

Duan J, Martinez M, Sanders AR, et al: Polymorphisms in the trace amine receptor 4 (TRAR4) gene on chromosome 6q23.2 are associated with susceptibility to schizophrenia. Am J Hum Genet 75:624–638, 2004

Egan MF, Goldberg TE, Kolachana BS, et al: Effect of COMT Val108/158 Met genotype on frontal lobe function and risk for schizophrenia. Proc Natl Acad Sci USA 98:6917–6922, 2001

Emamian ES, Hall D, Birnbaum MJ, et al: Convergent evidence for impaired AKT1-GSK3beta signaling in schizophrenia. Nat Genet 36: 131–137, 2004

Faraone SV, Matise T, Svrakic D, et al: Genome scan of European-American schizophrenia pedigrees: results of the NIMH Genetics Initiative and Millennium Consortium. Am J Med Genet Neuropsychiatr Genet 81:290–295, 1998

Farmer AE, McGuffin P, Gottesman II: Twin concordance for DSM-III schizophrenia: scrutinizing the validity of the definition. Arch Gen Psychiatry 44:634–640, 1987

Foley DL, Eaves LJ, Wormley B, et al: Childhood adversity, monoamine oxidase a genotype, and risk for conduct disorder. Arch Gen Psychiatry 61:738–744, 2004

Freedman R, Coon H, Myles-Worsley M, et al: Linkage of a neurophysiological deficit in schizophrenia to a chromosome 15 locus. Proc Natl Acad Sci USA 94:587–592, 1997

Funke B, Finn CT, Plocik AM, et al: Association of the DTNBP1 locus with schizophrenia in a U.S. population. Am J Hum Genet 75:891–898, 2004

Gault J, Logel J, Drebing C, et al: Mutation analysis of the α7 nicotinic acetylcholine receptor gene and its partial duplication in schizophrenia patients (abstract). Am J Hum Genet 65:A271, 1999

Gejman PV, Sanders AR, Badner JA, et al: Linkage analysis of schizophrenia to chromosome 15. Am J Med Genet 105:789–793, 2001

Gerber DJ, Hall D, Miyakawa T, et al: Evidence for association of schizophrenia with genetic variation in the 8p21.3 gene, PPP3CC, encoding the calcineurin gamma subunit. Proc Natl Acad Sci USA 100:8993–8998, 2003

Gill M, Vallada H, Collier D, et al: A combined analysis of D22S278 marker alleles in affected sib-pairs: support for a susceptibility locus for schizophrenia at chromosome 22q12. Am J Med Genet Neuropsychiatr Genet 67:40–45, 1996

Gottesman II: Schizophrenia genesis. New York, WH Freeman, 1991

Harrison PJ, Owen MJ: Genes for schizophrenia? Recent findings and their pathophysiological implications. Lancet 361:417–419, 2003

Hashimoto L, Habita C, Beressi JP, et al: Genetic mapping of a susceptibility locus for insulin-dependent diabetes mellitus on chromosome 11q. Nature 371:161–164, 1994

Heston LL: Psychiatric disorders in foster home reared children of schizophrenic mothers. Br J Psychiatry 112: 819–825, 1966

Hovatta I, Varilo T, Suvisaari J, et al: A genome-wide screen for schizophrenia genes in an isolated Finnish subpopulation suggesting multiple susceptibility loci. Am J Hum Genet 65:1114–1124, 1999

Hugot JP, Chamaillard M, Zouali H, et al: Association of NOD2 leucine-rich repeat variants with susceptibility to Crohn's disease. Nature 411:599–603, 2001

Kalsi G, Chen CH, Smyth C, et al: Genetic linkage analysis in an Icelandic/British sample fails to exclude the putative chromosome 13q14.1-q32 schizophrenia susceptibility locus (abstract). Am J Hum Genet 59:A388, 1996

Karayiorgou M, Morris MA, Morrow B, et al: Schizophrenia susceptibility associated with interstitial deletions of chromosome 22q11. Proc Natl Acad Sci USA 92:7612–7616, 1995

Kaufmann CA, Suarez B, Malaspina D, et al: NIMH Genetics Initiative Millennium Schizophrenia Consortium: Linkage analysis of African-American pedigrees. Am J Med Genet Neuropsychiatr Genet 81:282–289, 1998

Kendler KS: Schizophrenia genetics and dysbindin: a corner turned? Am J Psychiatry 161:1533–1536, 2004

Kendler KS, Diehl SR: The genetics of schizophrenia: a current, genetic-epidemiologic perspective. Schizophr Bull 19:261–285, 1993

Kendler KS, Gruenberg AM, Tsuang MT: A DSM-III family study of the nonschizophrenic psychotic disorders. Am J Psychiatry 143:1098–1105, 1986

Kendler KS, McGuire M, Gruenberg AM: The Roscommon Family Study, II: the risk of nonschizophrenic nonaffective psychoses in relatives. Arch Gen Psychiatry 50:645–652, 1993

Kendler KS, Straub RE, MacLean CJ, et al: Reflections on the evidence for a vulnerability locus for schizophrenia on chromosome 6p24–22. Am J Med Genet 67:124–126, 1996

Kendler KS, Kuhn JW, Prescott CA, et al: The interaction of stressful life events and a serotonin transporter polymorphism in the prediction of episodes of major depression: a replication. Arch Gen Psychiatry (in press)

Kety SS, Rosenthal D, Wender PH, et al: The types and prevalence of mental illness in the biological and adoptive families of adopted schizophrenics. J Psychiatr Res 6:345–362, 1968

Kety SS, Wender PH, Jacobsen B, et al: Mental illness in the biological and adoptive relatives of schizophrenic adoptees: replication of the Copenhagen study in the rest of Denmark. Arch Gen Psychiatry 51: 442–455, 1994

Kirov G, Ivanov D, Williams NM, et al: Strong evidence for association between the dystrobrevin binding protein 1 gene (DTNBP1) and schizophrenia in 488 parent-offspring trios from Bulgaria. Biol Psychiatry 55:971–975, 2004

Kohn Y, Danilovich E, Filon D, et al: Linkage disequilibrium in the DTNBP1 (dysbindin) gene region and on chromosome 1p36 among psychotic patients from a genetic isolate in Israel: findings from identity by descent haplotype sharing analysis. Am J Med Genet 128B:65–70, 2004

Korostishevsky M, Kaganovich M, Cholostoy A, et al: Is the G72/G30 locus associated with schizophrenia? Single nucleotide polymorphisms, haplotypes, and gene expression analysis. Biol Psychiatry 56:169–176, 2004

Laitinen T, Daly MJ, Rioux JD, et al: A susceptibility locus for asthma-related traits on chromosome 7 revealed by genome-wide scan in a founder population. Nat Genet 28:87–91, 2001

Lander E, Kruglyak L: Genetic dissection of complex traits: guidelines for interpreting and reporting linkage results. Nat Genet 11:241–247, 1995

Leonard S, Gault J, Moore T, et al: Further investigation of a chromosome 15 locus in schizophrenia: analysis of affected sibpairs from the NIMH Genetics Initiative. Am J Med Genet Neuropsychiatr Genet 81:308–312, 1998

Levinson DF, Wildenauer DB, Schwab SG, et al: Additional support for schizophrenia linkage on chromosomes 6 and 8: a multicenter study. Am J Med Genet Neuropsychiatr Genet 67:580–594, 1996

Levinson DF, Holmans P, Straub RE, et al: Multicenter linkage study of schizophrenia candidate regions on chromosomes 5q, 6q, 10p, and 13q: Schizophrenia Linkage Collaborative Group III. Am J Hum Genet 67:652–663, 2000

Levinson DF, Holmans PA, Laurent C, et al: No major schizophrenia locus detected on chromosome 1q in a large multicenter sample. Science 296:739–741, 2002

Lewis CM, Levinson DF, Wise LH, et al: Genome scan meta-analysis of schizophrenia and bipolar disorder, Part II: schizophrenia. Am J Hum Genet 73:34–48, 2003

Li T, Stefansson H, Gudfinnsson E, et al: Identification of a novel neuregulin 1 at-risk haplotype in Han schizophrenia Chinese patients, but no association with the Icelandic/Scottish risk haplotype. Mol Psychiatry 9:698–704, 2004

Lin MW, Curtis D, Williams N, et al: Suggestive evidence for linkage of schizophrenia to markers on chromosome 13q14.1-q32. Psychiatr Genet 5:117–126, 1995

Lin MW, Sham P, Hwu HG, et al: Suggestive evidence for linkage of schizophrenia to markers on chromosome 13 in Caucasian but not Oriental populations. Hum Genet 99:417–420, 1997

Lindholm E, Ekholm B, Balciuniene J, et al: Linkage analysis of a large Swedish kindred provides further support for a susceptibility locus for schizophrenia on chromosome 6p23. Am J Med Genet 88:369–377, 1999

Liu CM, Hwu HG, Lin MW, et al: Suggestive evidence for linkage of schizophrenia to markers at chromosome 15q13–14 in Taiwanese families. Am J Med Genet 105:658–661, 2001

Liu H, Heath SC, Sobin C, et al: Genetic variation at the 22q11 PRODH2/DGCR6 locus presents an unusual pattern and increases susceptibility to schizophrenia. Proc Natl Acad Sci USA 99:3717–3722, 2002

Martin ER, Monks SA, Warren LL, et al: A test for linkage and association in general pedigrees: The Pedigree Disequilibrium Test. Am J Hum Genet 67:146–154, 2000

Martinez M, Goldin LR, Cao Q, et al: Follow-up study on a susceptibility locus for schizophrenia on chromosome 6q. Am J Med Genet Neuropsychiatr Genet 88:337–343, 1999

Maziade M, Bissonnette L, Rouillard E, et al: 6p24–22 region and major psychoses in the Eastern Quebec population. Le Groupe IREP. Am J Med Genet 74:311–318, 1997

McGue M, Gottesman I, Rao DC: Resolving genetic models for the transmission of schizophrenia. Genet Epidemiol 2:99–110, 1985

Millar JK, Wilson-Annan JC, Anderson S, et al: Disruption of two novel genes by a translocation co-segregating with schizophrenia. Hum Mol Genet 9:1415–1423, 2000

Mirnics K, Middleton FA, Lewis DA, et al: Analysis of complex brain disorders with gene expression microarrays: schizophrenia as a disease of the synapse. Trends Neurosci 24:479–486, 2001

Moghaddam B: Bringing order to the glutamate chaos in schizophrenia. Neuron 40:881–884, 2003

Moises HW, Yang L, Kristbjarnarson H, et al: An international two-stage genome-wide search for schizophrenia susceptibility genes. Nat Genet 11:321–324, 1995

Morris DW, Rodgers A, McGhee KA, et al: Confirming RGS4 as a susceptibility gene for schizophrenia. Am J Med Genet 125B:50–53, 2004

Morton NE: Sequential tests for the detection of linkage. Am J Hum Genet 7:277–318, 1955

Murphy KC, Jones LA, Owen MJ: High rates of schizophrenia in adults with velo-cardio-facial syndrome. Arch Gen Psychiatry 56:940–945, 1999

Numakawa T, Yagasaki Y, Ishimoto T, et al: Evidence of novel neuronal functions of dysbindin, a susceptibility gene for schizophrenia. Hum Mol Genet 13:2699–2708, 2004

Ogura Y, Bonen DK, Inohara N, et al: A frameshift mutation in NOD2 associated with susceptibility to Crohn's disease. Nature 411:603–606, 2001

Polymeropoulos MH, Coon H, Byerley W, et al: Search for a schizophrenia susceptibility locus on human chromosome 22. Am J Med Genet 54:93–99, 1994

Prescott CA, Gottesman II: Genetically mediated vulnerability to schizophrenia. Psychiatr Clin North Am 16:245–267, 1993

Pulver AE, Karayiorgou M, Lasseter VK, et al: Follow-up of a report of a potential linkage for schizophrenia on chromosome 22q12-q13.1, Part 2. Am J Med Genet 54:44–50, 1994a

Pulver AE, Karayiorgou M, Wolyniec PS, et al: Sequential strategy to identify a susceptibility gene for schizophrenia: report of potential linkage on chromosome 22q12-q13.1, Part 1. Am J Med Genet 54:36–43, 1994b

Pulver AE, Nestadt G, Goldberg R, et al: Psychotic illness in patients diagnosed with velo-cardio-facial syndrome and their relatives. J Nerv Ment Dis 182:476–478, 1994c

Pulver AE, Lasseter VK, Kasch L, et al: Schizophrenia: a genome scan targets chromosomes 3p and 8p as potential sites of susceptibility genes. Am J Med Genet Neuropsychiatr Genet 60:252–260, 1995

Ray PN, Belfall B, Duff C, et al: Cloning of the breakpoint of an X;21 translocation associated with Duchenne muscular dystrophy. Nature 318:672–675, 1985

Riley BP, McGuffin P: Linkage and associated studies of schizophrenia. Am J Med Genet Semin Med Genet 97:23–44, 2000

Riley BP, Tahir E, Rajagopalan S, et al: A linkage study of the N-methyl-D-aspartate receptor subunit gene loci and schizophrenia in southern African Bantu-speaking families. Psychiatr Genet 7:57–74, 1997

Riley BP, Makoff A, Mogudi-Carter M, et al: Haplotype transmission disequilibrium and evidence for linkage of the CHRNA7 gene region to schizophrenia in southern African Bantu families. Am J Med Genet Neuropsychiatr Genet 96:196–201, 2000

Risch N: Linkage strategies for genetically complex traits, I: multilocus models. Am J Hum Genet 46:222–228, 1990

Sawcer S, Jones HB, Feakes R, et al: A genome screen in multiple sclerosis reveals susceptibility loci on chromosome 6p21 and 17q22. Nat Genet 13:464–468, 1996

Schumacher J, Jamra RA, Freudenberg J, et al: Examination of G72 and D-amino-acid oxidase as genetic risk factors for schizophrenia and bipolar affective disorder. Mol Psychiatry 9:203–207, 2004

Schwab SG, Albus M, Hallmayer J, et al: Evaluation of a susceptibility gene for schizophrenia on chromosome 6p by multipoint affected sib-pair linkage analysis. Nat Genet 11:325–327, 1995

Schwab SG, Eckstein GN, Hallmayer J, et al: Evidence suggestive of a locus on chromosome 5q31 contributing to susceptibility for schizophrenia in German and Israeli families by multipoint affected sib-pair linkage analysis. Mol Psychiatry 2:156–160, 1997

Schwab SG, Hallmayer J, Albus M, et al: Further evidence for a susceptibility locus on chromosome 10p14-p11 in 72 families with schizophrenia by nonparametric linkage analysis. Am J Med Genet Neuropsychiatr Genet 81:302–307, 1998

Schwab SG, Knapp M, Mondabon S, et al: Support for association of schizophrenia with genetic variation in the 6p22.3 gene, dysbindin, in sib-pair families with linkage and in an additional sample of triad families. Am J Hum Genet 72:185–190, 2003

Shaw SH, Kelly M, Smith AB, et al: A genome-wide search for schizophrenia susceptibility genes. Am J Med Genet Neuropsychiatr Genet 81:364–376, 1998

Sherrington R, Brynjolfsson J, Petursson H, et al: Localization of a susceptibility locus for schizophrenia on chromosome 5. Nature 336:164–167, 1988

Shifman S, Bronstein M, Sternfeld M, et al: A highly significant association between a COMT haplotype and schizophrenia. Am J Hum Genet 71:1296–1302, 2002

Spielman RS, Ewens WJ: The TDT and other family based tests for linkage disequilibrium and association. Am J Hum Genet 59:983–989, 1996

Stefansson H, Sigurdsson E, Steinthorsdottir V, et al: Neuregulin 1 and susceptibility to schizophrenia. Am J Hum Genet 71:877–892, 2002

Stefansson H, Sarginson J, Kong A, et al: Association of neuregulin 1 with schizophrenia confirmed in a Scottish population. Am J Hum Genet 72: 83–87, 2003

Straub RE, MacLean CJ, O'Neill FA, et al: A potential vulnerability locus for schizophrenia on chromosome 6p24–22: evidence for genetic heterogeneity. Nature Genetics 11:287–293, 1995

Straub RE, MacLean CJ, O'Neill FA, et al: Support for a possible schizophrenia vulnerability locus in region 5q22–31 in Irish families. Mol Psychiatry 2:148–155, 1997

Straub RE, MacLean CJ, Martin RB, et al: A schizophrenia locus may be located in region 10p15-p11. Am J Med Genet Neuropsychiatr Genet 81:296–301, 1998

Straub RE, Jiang Y, MacLean CJ, et al: Genetic variation in the 6p22.3 gene DTNBP1, the human ortholog of mouse dysbindin, is associated with schizophrenia. Am J Hum Genet 71:337–348, 2002

Sullivan PF, Kendler KS, Neale MC: Schizophrenia as a complex trait: evidence from a meta-analysis of twin studies. Arch Gen Psychiatry 60:1187–1192, 2003

Talbot K, Eidem WL, Tinsley CL, et al: Dysbindin-1 is reduced in intrinsic, glutamatergic terminals of the hippocampal formation in schizophrenia. J Clin Invest 113:1353–1363, 2004

Tang JX, Zhou J, Fan JB, et al: Family based association study of DTNBP1 in 6p22.3 and schizophrenia. Mol Psychiatry 8:717–718, 2003

Tang JX, Chen WY, He G, et al: Polymorphisms within 5' end of the neuregulin 1 gene are genetically associated with schizophrenia in the Chinese population. Mol Psychiatry 9:11–12, 2004

Tienari P: Interaction between genetic vulnerability and family environment: the Finnish Adoptive Family Study of Schizophrenia. Acta Psychiatr Scand 84:460–465, 1991

Tienari P, Wynne LC, Sorri A, et al: Genotype-environment interaction in schizophrenia-spectrum disorder: long-term follow-up study of Finnish adoptees. Br J Psychiatry 184:216–222, 2004

Tsuang DW, Skol AD, Faraone SV, et al: Examination of genetic linkage of chromosome 15 to schizophrenia in a large Veterans Affairs Cooperative study sample. Am J Med Genet 105:662–668, 2001

Van Den Bogaert A, Schumacher J, Schulze TG, et al: The DTNBP1 (dysbindin) gene contributes to schizophrenia, depending on family history of the disease. Am J Hum Genet 73:1438–1443, 2003

van den Oord E, Sullivan PF, Chen X., et al: Identification of a high risk haplotype for the dystrobrevin binding protein 1 (DTNBP1) gene in the Irish study of high density schizophrenia families. Mol Psychiatry 8:499–510, 2003

Vionnet N, Hani E, Dupont S, et al: Genomewide search for type 2 diabetes-susceptibility genes in French whites: evidence for a novel susceptibility locus for early onset diabetes on chromosome 3q27-qter and independent replication of a type 2-diabetes locus on chromosome 1q21-q24. Am J Hum Genet 67:1470–1480, 2000

Wang X, He G, Gu N, et al: Association of G72/G30 with schizophrenia in the Chinese population. Biochem Biophys Res Commun 319:1281–1286, 2004

Weickert CS, Straub R, McClintock B, et al: Human dysbindin (DTNBP1) gene expression in normal brain and in schizophrenic prefrontal cortex and midbrain. Arch Gen Psychiatry 61:544–555, 2004

Williams NM, Preece A, Spurlock G, et al: Support for genetic variation in neuregulin 1 and susceptibility to schizophrenia. Mol Psychiatry 8:485–487, 2003

Williams NM, Preece A, Morris DW, et al: Identification in 2 independent samples of a novel schizophrenia risk haplotype of the dystrobrevin binding protein gene (DTNBP1). Arch Gen Psychiatry 61:336–344, 2004a

Williams NM, Preece A, Spurlock G, et al: Support for RGS4 as a susceptibility gene for schizophrenia. Biol Psychiatry 55:192–195, 2004b

Wiltshire S, Hattersley AT, Hitman GA, et al: A genomewide scan for loci predisposing to type 2 diabetes in a UK population (the Diabetes UK Warren 2 Repository): analysis of 573 pedigrees provides independent replication of a susceptibility locus on chromosome 1q. Am J Hum Genet 69:553–569, 2001

Xu J, Pato MT, Torre CD, et al: Evidence for linkage disequilibrium between the alpha7-nicotinic receptor gene (CHRNA7) locus and schizophrenia in Azorean families. Am J Med Genet 105:669–674, 2001

Yang JZ, Si TM, Ruan Y, et al: Association study of neuregulin 1 gene with schizophrenia. Mol Psychiatry 8:706–709, 2003

Zhao X, Shi Y, Tang J, et al: A case control and family based association study of the neuregulin1 gene and schizophrenia. J Med Genet 41:31–34, 2004

Chapter 4

Genetics of Anxiety Disorders

John M. Hettema, M.D., Ph.D.

In this chapter, we review the available human data on genetic factors that contribute to the liability for developing anxiety disorders (ADs). With lifetime prevalence of ADs as a group estimated to be as high as 25% (Kessler et al. 1994), they are among the most common of the psychiatric disorders. They possess substantial lifetime comorbidity with each other and with other psychiatric conditions (Noyes and Hoehn-Saric 1998), most notably mood disorders (Maser and Cloninger 1990). They can be significantly disabling, carrying a burden of impairment comparable to that of chronic "medical" disorders, such as diabetes.

A long history of family studies has sought to determine whether ADs aggregate in families. As there are no published adoption studies of ADs, researchers have relied on twin studies to disentangle the effects of genetics and environment and to estimate their heritability. Our group recently published a meta-analysis to summarize findings across family and twin studies of ADs (Hettema et al. 2001a). We restricted our selection of studies to include only those that 1) used operationalized diagnostic criteria; 2) systematically selected (or more technically, "ascertained") and 3) directly interviewed the majority of subjects (thus excluding family history studies); 4) performed the diagnostic assessment of relatives blind to proband affection status; and 5) for the family studies, included a control group. We used the meta-analysis to evaluate consistency between apparently differing results by testing for homogeneity across studies, and to combine data from multiple primary studies to provide more reliable, precise, and less biased aggregate estimates of familial risk and heritability. In the family studies, we report the odds ratio (OR) as the measure of association between illness in the selected subject ("proband") and in first-degree relatives. An OR greater than 1.0 reflects the increased risk of illness in a relative of an affected proband compared to relatives of unaffected ("control") probands, suggesting familial aggregation of the condition. For twin studies, probandwise concordance estimates the risk in the co-twin of an affected twin, while heritability here estimates the proportion of variance for the trait or disorder that is accounted for by genetics.

Linkage and association analyses have begun to investigate the molecular underpinnings of the genetic epidemiological findings. We summarize the extant literature on molecular genetics of the ADs, keeping in mind that most of the findings are early, tentative, and await replication.

Finally, although the genetics of anxiety symptoms, anxiety-related traits, and animal models of fear and anxiety have received much research attention, these topics are outside the scope of this review. We address their role in the final section of this chapter when we consider future directions.

Panic Disorder

Family Studies

Five family studies of panic disorder (PD), all from clinical populations, met the inclusion criteria for the meta-analysis (Table 4–1). All five studies support the familial aggregation of PD (OR > 1.0). In addition, the findings of a secondary analysis of the Horwath et al. (1995) data suggest that early-onset PD in the proband is associated with higher familial risk (Goldstein et al. 1997). The results of our meta-analysis show a highly significant association between PD in the proband and PD in first-degree relatives. The summary OR across the five studies was 5.0 (95% CI: 3.0–8.2), strongly supporting a familial component in liability to PD. The unadjusted aggregate risk across the studies, based on 1,356 total first-degree relatives of PD probands, was 10.0%, compared with 2.1% in 1,187 control relatives.

Table 4–1. Family studies of panic disorder (PD) and panic disorder with or without agoraphobia (PDA)

Study	Proband's diagnosis	Cases				Controls				OR (95% CI)
		Source	N_P	N_R	MR^a	Source	N_P	N_R	MR^a	
Noyes et al. 1986	PD (DSM-III)	Clinical	40	241	17.3	Nonanxious	20	113	4.2	4.8 (1.6–13.8)
Mendlewicz et al. 1993	PD (DSM-III)	Clinical	25	122	13.2	NMI	25	130	0.9	15.6 (2.0–121)
Maier et al. 1993	PDA (DSM-III-R)	Clinical	40	174	7.9	Unscreened GP	80	309	2.3	3.6 (1.3–10.2)
Horwath et al. 1995	PDA (DSM-III-R)	Clinical	107	583	11.0	GP NMI	45	255	1.8	6.7 (2.1–21.7)
Fyer et al. 1996	PDA (DSM-III-R)	Clinical	79	220	9.5	NMI	77	231	3	3.4 (1.4–8.1)
						Mantel-Haenszel summary OR				5.0 (3.0–8.2)

Note. CI=confidence interval; GP=general population; MR=morbidity risk; NMI=never mentally ill; N_P=number of probands; N_R=number of first-degree relatives; OR=odds ratio.
[a]MR=morbidity risk (%) in first-degree relatives: uncorrected (Fyer et al. 1996) and age-corrected by Kaplan-Meier analysis (Horwath et al. 1995) or Strömgren method for others.

Source. Reprinted from Hettema JM, Neale MC, Kendler KS: "A Review and Meta-analysis of the Genetic Epidemiology of Anxiety Disorders." *American Journal of Psychiatry* 158:1568–1578, 2001. Copyright 2001, American Psychiatric Association. Used with permission.

Twin Studies

While several smaller twin studies found tentative evidence suggesting that the etiological basis for PD is at least, in part, genetic, the two largest sources of twin data for PD are the population-based Virginia Adult Twin Study of Psychiatric and Substance Use Disorders (VATSPSUD), and the Vietnam Era Twin (VET) Registry. The former consists of approximately 6,000 twins from male and female same-sex and opposite-sex pairs, while the latter is of comparable size but contains only male twins who served during the Vietnam War. The size of these samples permits the use of structural equation modeling to assess the relative contributions of additive genetics, common family environment, and individual specific environment to the liability of PD. However, even in these samples, diagnostic criteria were broadened to overcome power limitations introduced by the relatively low prevalence of PD (2%–3%) in the general population.

The VATSPSUD examined panic syndromes in two studies of same-sex female (Kendler et al. 1993) and same-sex male and opposite-sex pairs (Kendler et al. 2001a), respectively, while the VET study analyzed the relationship between panic and generalized anxiety syndromes (Scherrer et al. 2000). Analyses from both samples are consistent in attributing 30%–40% of the variance in liability of PD to genetic risk factors, with the remainder of the variance deriving from individual specific environment. They do not support a significant role for common family environment in the etiology of PD, suggesting that the basis for familial aggregation of PD is genetic in origin. In addition, the combined male-female analysis from the VATSPSUD found no evidence that genetic risk factors differ between men and women.

Molecular Genetic Studies

Three multifamily, genomewide linkage analyses specific to PD and one examining a broader range of ADs, with PD as the primary focus, have been published. The first, from the Columbia University group, was performed in 23 high-density families defined as having at least three affected relatives with PD and agoraphobia in two different generations (Knowles et al. 1998). In their first-pass genome scan using both parametric linkage analysis within kindreds and nonparametric sib-pair linkage analysis, Knowles et al. (1998) reported six markers with LOD (logarithm of the odds) scores between 1.0 and 2.0 on chromosomes 1p, 20p (dominant model) and 7p, 17p, 20q, X/Y (recessive model)—scores that fall substantially short of the threshold LOD score of 3.3 required for definite linkage to a complex trait like PD. That group reported a second linkage analysis in 60 multiplex pedigrees of a broad syndrome that included PD, bladder problems, severe headaches, mitral valve prolapse, and thyroid conditions. These authors found significant linkage on chromosomes 13q, and possibly 22, under a dominant genetic model (Hamilton et al. 2003).

A second genomewide linkage scan for PD was performed by the University of Iowa group in 23 multiplex families (Crowe et al. 2001). They reported a maximum LOD score of 2.23 on chromosome 7p15, close to the region of the peak LOD score (1.71) from the Knowles et al. study above. A reanalysis of these data using a Bayesian approach obtained an 80% probability of linkage to marker D16S749 in that region (Logue et al. 2003).

The third group, from Yale University, reported the results of a linkage analysis for PD and agoraphobia phenotypes in a set of 20 pedigrees (Gelernter et al. 2001). They identified two regions with suggestive linkage to PD. The first, with a LOD score of 2.04 on chromosome 1, was close to a region of LOD score 1.1 in the Crowe et al. study. The second, with a LOD score of 2.01 on chromosome 11, occurred at the CCKBR marker, one of the a priori candidate regions genotyped in this analysis (see below).

Finally, a linkage study was performed on a set of 25 families, which had at least one member affected with PD, selected from a larger sample of 62 families in the Icelandic population affected with a broad range of ADs (Thorgeirsson et al. 2003). Family members were considered "affected" in the linkage analysis if they were diagnosed with any DSM-III-R or ICD-10 anxiety disorders. Of the 60 affected relative pairs included in the analysis, there were 3 pairs in which both members had PD, 41 pairs in which one had PD and the other a separate AD, and 16 pairs in which the subjects had other ADs but not PD. The highest LOD score was 4.18, which was obtained for a region on chromosome 9, corresponding to a genomewide significance level of $P < 0.05$. LOD scores between 1.0 and 2.0 were observed on chromosomes 3, 4, 15, 18, and X.

A large number of candidate-gene association studies of PD have been published. As most of these are single studies of specific genes with negative results, we focus here on those that show preliminary promise for association with PD. The candidate biological system that has probably received the most attention is that of the neuropeptide cholecystokinin (CCK). The CCK tetrapeptide, CCK-4, can induce panic attacks in both healthy subjects and patients with PD, with the latter showing enhanced sensitivity to its panicogenic effects (Bradwejn et al. 1991). However, conflicting evidence from association analyses performed on different samples makes the role of CCK in the pathophysiology of PD unclear at present.

Catechol-O-methyltransferase (COMT), the enzyme involved in the inactivation of catecholamines, has been implicated in pathological anxiety states from animal and clinical studies. The gene (*COMT*) is located on chromosome 22 and possesses an allelic variation (472G/A-Val/Met) that produces a three- to fourfold difference in activity level of COMT enzymatic activity. A case-control association study in a Korean sample of 51 PD patients and 45 controls reported a significant association between PD and the low-activity allele (Woo et al. 2002). The Columbia University group analyzed COMT for linkage and association with PD in their family-based sample of 70 PD pedigrees and 83 parent-offspring triads (Hamilton et al. 2002). They found significant linkage for several polymorphisms, including the 472G/A single-nucleotide polymorphism (SNP), as well as significant association for several haplotypes made up of combinations of the polymorphisms, although, unlike the Korean study, their study suggested that the high-activity allele may be associated with PD. Thus, COMT, or a gene in linkage disequilibrium with it, may increase the liability for developing PD.

The adenosine system has also been suggested as a candidate neural substrate involved in PD. Caffeine, like CCK-4, precipitates panic attacks in susceptible individuals and acts as an antagonist at the adenosine receptors. In an early study in a German sample of 89 patients and matched controls, a significant association was reported between a silent SNP in the coding region of the adenosine A2a receptor gene and PD (Deckert et al. 1998). This finding has been supported by linkage and family-based association analyses in the large sample from the Columbia University group (Hamilton et al. 2004). However, no association was found for this polymorphism in a sample of Japanese PD patients, possibly because of ethnic differences in allele frequencies between the two populations (Yamada et al. 2001). This suggests that the adenosine A2a receptor gene may be implicated in the pathophysiology of PD in some, but not all, ethnic groups.

Another interesting candidate gene that has been examined in PD is the monoamine oxidase–A (MAO-A) gene, involved primarily in the intracellular enzymatic degradation of serotonin and norepinephrine. However, one positive report of association and two negative reports make this a less likely candidate than originally hypothesized. Several as yet unreplicated reports using small case-control samples in a Japanese population provide tentative evidence of associations between PD and other serotonin-related genes.

Summary

PD is a syndrome with moderate familial aggregation and heritability. The overall lifetime morbidity risk in first-degree relatives of PD patients is almost eight times that in relatives of healthy individuals, with a possible higher risk in relatives of persons with early-onset cases. Linkage studies are just beginning to converge on genomic loci that likely contribute to this risk, while association studies provide tentative evidence for specific involvement of the COMT gene and the adenosine A2a receptor gene in PD.

Generalized Anxiety Disorder

Family Studies

Only one published family study of generalized anxiety disorder (GAD) met all of the inclusion criteria from our meta-analysis

(Mendlewicz et al. 1993). That study, cited in the previous section on PD, compared the morbidity risk of several ADs in the first-degree relatives of four age- and sex-matched proband groups from a German clinical sample: those with PD, GAD, or major depressive disorder (MDD), and healthy controls. The age-corrected morbidity risk for GAD was higher in relatives of GAD probands (8.9%±1.2%) compared with relatives of PD (4.0%±0.8%), MDD (4.9%±0.9%), and control probands (1.9%±0.5%), although these differences did not reach statistical significance as a group. When only the GAD and control proband groups were compared, the OR for GAD was 5.0 (95% CI [confidence interval]: 1.0–24.3).

We included one additional study for comparison, that of Noyes et al. (1987), which met all the criteria except blind assessment. This analysis extended the family study of PD cited in the previous section (Noyes et al. 1986) by comparing the relatives of generalized anxiety, panic, agoraphobic, and healthy probands, this time for a range of anxiety disorders as well as alcohol and affective disorders. Again, the rates of GAD were higher in the relatives of GAD compared with the other three proband groups, with a significant GAD-control proband difference (19.5% versus 3.5%, $\chi^2=14.37$, $df=1$, $P<.001$). The OR for GAD in GAD versus control probands was 6.6 (95% CI: 2.2–19.7). Both studies support the familial aggregation of GAD, and together they show a significant association between GAD in the proband and in their first-degree relatives, with a summary OR of 6.08 (95% CI: 2.5–14.9).

Twin Studies

A Norwegian study of 81 adult twins with DSM-III-R anxiety disorders reported that GAD was four times more frequent in monozygotic (MZ) than in dizygotic (DZ) co-twins of GAD probands (3/5 vs. 1/7, not significant) (Skre et al. 1993). Both the VATSPSUD and the VET Registry assessed GAD in their samples, although both also used broadened GAD-like syndromes to obtain sufficient power for modeling. As in the PD analyses, the VATSPSUD examined GAD syndromes in two separate studies: the first in same-sex female twin pairs (Kendler et al. 1992a) and the second in same-sex male and female and opposite-sex pairs (Hettema et al. 2001b). The VET Registry study for PD and GAD in males is that cited earlier in the discussion of PD (Scherrer et al. 2000). Although the best-fitting model varied somewhat across syndromic definitions and interview waves of the VATSPSUD (the latter likely due to poor reliability of GAD), the overall picture suggests that GAD may have only modest heritability (15%–30%) with an uncertain but likely smaller role for common family environment in its familial aggregation. The VET Registry study found a heritability of 38%. When the findings from both samples were combined in a meta-analytic fashion, the best-fit model predicted that 31.6% (95% CI: 24%–39%) of the variance for liability to developing GAD was attributable to additive genetics, and no significant gender differences were detected. The model also estimated a small role for common familial (shared) environment in the females only, with the remaining variance attributable to individual specific environment.

Molecular Genetic Studies

There are currently no published linkage studies for GAD. A handful of small association studies have examined candidate genes in GAD, with unreplicated positive associations reported thus far for the dopamine transporter gene, the serotonin transporter gene, and the MAO-A gene. Caution is warranted in interpreting the significance of these findings until they are confirmed in larger, independent samples.

Summary

Although there is less available evidence for GAD than for PD because of the fewer available studies, the data support familial aggregation of GAD, and this is likely due to genetics rather than to family environment. The status of the molecular genetics of GAD is still too premature to support the involvement of any specific genetic loci in its etiology.

Phobias

Family Studies

Given the scarcity of genetic studies of the phobia subtypes, specific phobias, social phobia, and agoraphobia will be grouped together in this section. Four family studies of phobias met criteria for inclusion in the meta-analysis (Table 4–2). All studies individually support the familial aggregation of phobias. The OR values are similar across all studies except for that of Stein et al. 1998; however, they are all statistically consistent with one another. The results of the meta-analysis show that there is a highly significant association between a phobia in the proband and in first-degree relatives, with a summary OR of 4.07 (95% CI: 2.7–6.1) that strongly supports increased familial risk for phobic disorders.

Twin Studies

In his early studies of Norwegian twins, Torgersen found that genetic factors played a role in several categories of common phobic fears (Torgersen 1979). A small number of subsequent twin studies support the hypothesis of a genetic component underlying self-report fear symptoms. The only large, adult twin sample that has examined the genetics of phobias is the VATSPSUD. Although varying somewhat by the analysis applied to the sample, the preponderance of evidence suggests that genetics is primarily responsible for twin resemblance for agoraphobia, social phobia, and specific phobia subtypes, with little or no role for common familial environmental factors shared by the twins (Kendler et al. 1992b, 2000; Neale et al. 1994). Although the VATSPSUD has been the only large, adult twin sample in which a comprehensive study of the phobias has been made, the data from this sample support the familial aggregation seen in the family studies, with genetics explaining from one-third to two-thirds of individual differences for fears and phobias, depending on the analysis and type of phobia.

Molecular Genetic Studies

Currently, there are two published linkage studies for phobias, both from a research group at Yale University. The first included 129 subjects from 14 pedigrees in which two or more family members were affected by simple phobia (a subgroup of those families originally ascertained for PD described previously). That

Table 4–2. Family studies of simple (specific) phobias (P), social phobia (SP), generalized social phobia (GSP), and agoraphobia (AG)

Study	Proband's diagnosis	Cases				Controls				
		Source	N_P	N_R	MR[a]	Source	N_P	N_R	MR[a]	OR (95% CI)
Noyes et al. 1986	AG (DSM-III)	Clinical	40	241	11.6	Nonanxious	20	113	4.2	3.0 (1.0–8.9)
Fyer et al. 1995	P (DSM-III-R)	Clinical	15	49	31	NMI	77	231	9	4.4 (2.1–9.4)
	AG (DSM-III-R)	Clinical	49	131	10	NMI	77	231	3	3.5 (1.4–9.1)
Mannuzza et al. 1995	GSP (DSM-III-R)	Clinical	33	96	16	NMI	77	380	6	2.9 (1.4–5.7)
Stein et al. 1998	GSP (DSM-IV)	Clinical	23	106	26.4	NMI	24	74	2.7	12.9 (2.9–56.2)
						Mantel-Haenszel summary OR				4.1 (2.7–6.1)

Note. CI=confidence interval; NMI=never mentally ill; N_P=number of probands; N_R = number of first-degree relatives; OR=odds ratio. [a]MR=morbidity risk (%) in first-degree relatives: age-corrected (Strömgren method) by Noyes Jr et al. 1986 only; all others are uncorrected rates.

Source. Reprinted from Hettema JM, Neale MC, Kendler KS: "A Review and Meta-Analysis of the Genetic Epidemiology of Anxiety Disorders." *American Journal of Psychiatry* 158:1568–1578, 2001. Copyright 2001, American Psychiatric Association. Used with permission.

study reported significant linkage (LOD scores>3.0) on chromosome 14 and suggestive linkage (LOD>2.0) on chromosome 8 under various models of transmission (Gelernter et al. 2003). In mostly the same set of families, they also reported a finding of suggestive linkage of a region on chromosome 16 to social phobia (Gelernter et al. 2004). Prior to these studies, several serotonin and dopamine candidate genes had been excluded for linkage to social phobia.

Summary

Phobias tend to aggregate in families, with an OR of about 4.0, an odds ratio comparable to those for PD and GAD, which have historically been considered more "biological." Despite suggestions by social learning theory of the importance of vicarious learning of phobic fears from family members in the etiology of phobias, the twin data show that familial aggregation stems largely from genetic factors versus common environmental factors. Although some of the family study data predict familial aggregation that is specific to phobia subtypes, the twin data support the hypothesis of a nonspecific "inherited phobia proneness." The molecular genetics of phobias is still in its early stages.

Obsessive-Compulsive Disorder

Family Studies

Four family studies of obsessive-compulsive disorder (OCD) met our inclusion criteria, and another met all except the crtierion of blind assessment. The details of these five studies treated in the meta-analysis are listed in Table 4–3. It should be noted that there are substantial differences in methodology between the studies, the discussion of which is outside the scope of this review. Separately, these five family studies provide mixed support for familial aggregation of OCD, since for the first three the OR did not significantly differ from 1.0. Taken together, however, there is a highly significant association between OCD in the proband and OCD in first-degree relatives (summary OR statistic=25.1, $df=1$, $P<.0001$). The summary OR across the five studies is 4.0 (95% CI:

2.2–7.1), supporting the familial aggregation of OCD. The unadjusted aggregate risk based on 1,209 total first-degree relatives of OCD probands equals 8.2% versus 2.0% in 746 control relatives. Several other family studies that did not meet our inclusion criteria generally support these findings.

Some interesting corollary findings were reported in these studies. Pauls et al. (1995) performed a secondary analysis that examined whether age at onset was related to risk among relatives. They found an approximately twofold higher risk of OCD among relatives of probands with early (<18 years) age at onset than among relatives of probands with later onset. This finding was confirmed by similar results in the Nestadt et al. 2000 study as well as by findings in one of the family studies not included in Table 4–3 (Bellodi et al. 1992). Thus, age at onset appears to increase familial risk for OCD. Furthermore, most studies suggest that, in addition to fully syndromic OCD, a milder, subthreshold form of obsessive-compulsive symptomatology is seen with increased frequency in relatives of OCD probands.

Twin Studies

There have only been a handful of twin studies of OCD, and we could not identify any that met our inclusion criteria. The following discussion is therefore limited to the few existing twin studies of obsessive-compulsive symptoms or features. Rasmussen and Tsuang (1986) reviewed early literature reports of twins with OCD. Most of these were case studies lacking data for DZ twins, but an overall MZ concordance rate of 63% was reported. A small study in 15 MZ and 15 twin DZ pairs reported concordance rates for obsessive-compulsive symptoms or features of 87% and 47%, respectively, but only 33% and 7% for episodes requiring treatment (Carey and Gottesman 1981). Clifford et al. (1984) analyzed obsessive-compulsive traits and symptoms assessed by the Leyton Obsessional Inventory in 419 complete pairs from a London-based volunteer twin registry. They reported heritability estimates of 44% for obsessive-compulsive traits and 47% for symptoms, with the remainder of the variance for these measures explained by a nonshared environment. In the largest study to date, self-reported obsessive and compulsive symptoms from the Padua Inventory

Table 4–3. Family studies of OCD

Study	Diagnostic criteria	Cases					Controls				
		Blind	Source	N_P	N_R	MR^a	Source	N_P	N_R	MR^a	OR (95% CI)
McKeon and Murray 1987	ICD/RDC	N	Clinical	50	149	0.7	NMI surgical	50	151	0.7	1.0 (.06–16.3)
Black et al. 1992	DSM-III	Y	Clinical	32	120	2.6	NMI volunteers	33	129	2.4	1.1 (.21–5.4)
Fyer et al. 1993[b]; Rasmussen 1993	DSM-III	Y	Clinical	50	148	7.0	NMI	—	—	2.0	3.9 (.49–31.9)
Pauls et al. 1995	DSM-III-R	Y	Clinical	100	466	10.3	NMI volunteers	33	113	1.9	5.9 (1.4–24.8)
Nestadt et al. 2000	DSM-IV	Y	Clinical	80	326	11.7	GP	73	297	2.7	4.8 (2.2–10.3)
							Mantel-Haenszel summary OR				4.0 (2.2–7.1)

Note. CI=confidence interval; ICD=International Classification of Diseases (1975); NMI=never mentally ill; N_P=number of probands; N_R=number of first-degree relatives; OR=odds ratio; RDC=Research Diagnostic Criteria (1978).
[a]MR=morbidity risk (%) in first-degree relatives: uncorrected (McKeon and Murray 1987, Fyer et al. 1993, and Nestadt et al. 2000); age-corrected by Strömgren method (Black et al. 1992) or survival analysis (Pauls et al. 1995).
[b]Preliminary results (private communication).
Source. Reprinted from Hettema JM, Neale MC, Kendler KS: "A Review and Meta-analysis of the Genetic Epidemiology of Anxiety Disorders." *American Journal of Psychiatry* 158:1568–1578, 2001. Copyright 2001, American Psychiatric Association. Used with permission.

were examined in 1,054 female twins from the VATSPSUD (Jonnal et al. 2000). Factor analysis identified two major factors accounting for 62% of the variance that appeared to roughly correspond to obsessions and compulsions, respectively. These factors had heritabilities of 33% and 26%, respectively, with a genetic correlation of +0.53 between them. While these studies can provide insight into the potential genetic basis of variables that are related to the OCD phenotype, speculations on the common genetic basis between these variables and syndromic OCD are outside of the scope of this review.

Molecular Genetic Studies

Two published genomewide linkage studies of OCD currently exist. The first examined the obsessive-compulsive symptom of hoarding in a cohort of 77 sibling pairs identified because they were concordant for Gilles de la Tourette syndrome (Zhang et al. 2002). The analysis identified several potential regions (4q, 5q, and 17q) with significant linkage to this phenotype. The second linkage scan was performed in 66 subjects from seven families ascertained through pediatric (i.e., early onset) OCD probands (Hanna et al. 2002). That analysis provided suggestive evidence for linkage on 9p (LOD=~2.0) and identified two other regions on 6p and 19q with LOD scores between 1.0 and 2.0. The findings on 9p were supported by the Johns Hopkins group in a follow-up linkage study targeting this region (Willour et al. 2004).

As in PD, a large number of (mostly nonreplicated) candidate-gene association studies of OCD have been published. These have focused primarily on the serotonergic and dopaminergic systems, which have been hypothesized to play a role in the pathogenesis of this disorder on the basis of animal, biological, imaging, and pharmacological studies. Given that genes from these two neurotransmitter systems make up the "usual suspects" for neuropsychiatric illness, it is not surprising that many of the same genes have been examined in OCD as in PD above. For example, the COMT 472G/A-Val/Met polymorphism has been studied by several groups using both case-control and family-based association methods, with mixed results. A recent meta-analysis (Azzam and Mathews 2003) examined the data across these studies, concluding that insufficient evidence exists to support an association between COMT and OCD.

The serotonin transporter in general, because of its role in the action of serotonin reuptake inhibitor (SRI) antidepressants used to treat OCD, and the SLC6A4 polymorphism in the gene's upstream regulatory region (5-HTTLPR) in particular have received much attention for OCD and related disorders—especially since the initial report of the association of this polymorphism with anxiety-related traits (Lesch et al. 1996). However, the association studies with negative findings currently outnumber the positive ones, leaving insufficient evidence to support an association between this serotonin transporter polymorphism and OCD.

Two other serotonin genes, the serotonin$_{2A}$ receptor gene (5HT2A) and the serotonin$_{1D}$ β autoreceptor gene (5HT1Dβ), have also been examined by several groups for possible association with OCD. Positive reports of association in three small, independent, population-based samples provide tentative evidence for a role of 5HT2A in the etiology of OCD, warranting further investigation in larger, preferably family-based samples. However, the conflicting findings of these reports make support for association of 5HT1Dβ with OCD less convincing.

Genes for various components of the dopaminergic system (dopamine transporter, dopamine receptor types 2, 3, and 4) have been investigated for association with OCD. The only replicated association was for a 48-bp repeat in exon III of the dopamine type 4 receptor gene (DRD4) reported by the Toronto group in a Canadian sample of 63 OCD patients and 55 matched controls, with only a marginally significant P value (0.021; uncorrected for multiple testing) (Billett et al. 1998). This finding was replicated in a family-based and case-control sample, whereas two other case-control studies did not find an association between this gene and OCD.

Finally, two groups have reported an association between the MAO-A gene and OCD. The first study, using both a case-control sample and a family-based analysis in 51 OCD trios, reported a difference in allelic frequencies for the EcoRV polymorphism for OCD patients (Camarena et al. 2001). The second study reported an association between a different MAO-A polymorphism and OCD in males from a sample of 110 families with OCD (Karayiorgou et al.

1999). Although replication in larger samples is warranted, there is evidence suggesting a role for the MAO-A gene in OCD.

Summary

Family study data support the familial aggregation of OCD, particularly in early-onset cases. Twin data from large, population-based samples adequately assessed for this complex phenotype are lacking, but the available data are suggestive of the importance of genetic risk factors in OCD. Although linkage and association studies for OCD are under way, it is too early to predict which specific genes are clearly implicated in its etiology.

Posttraumatic Stress Disorder

Family Studies

The study of the genetics of posttraumatic stress disorder (PTSD) is complicated by the requirement of a specific environmental exposure in the diagnosis of this disorder. The classification of a subject as not carrying an increased risk for PTSD (i.e., "healthy") is predicated on the condition that he or she is unaffected only *after* experiencing a significant trauma, providing unique challenges to the sample selection. However, a handful of published family studies exist, mostly examining general psychopathology in the relatives of PTSD probands to identify correlated familial risk factors. For example, in an urban sample of 1,007 young adults, Breslau et al. (1991) examined the risk factors for exposure to trauma and for development of PTSD given that exposure occurred, finding that neuroticism and familial anxiety, among other factors, increased the risk for developing PTSD after the experience of a traumatic event. Overall, a family history of either ADs or depressive disorders or both may increase an individual's risk for developing PTSD after experiencing a significant trauma.

Twin Studies

Two published twin studies of PTSD currently exist. The first, from the VET Registry, analyzed the genetic and environmental risk factors for 15 self-reported symptoms of PTSD from the reexperiencing, avoidance, and hyperarousal clusters as well as trauma exposure in 4,042 complete male twin pairs (True et al. 1993). The MZ twin correlations were higher than the DZ twin correlations for all of the symptoms and for trauma exposure, suggesting genes may increase the risk of experiencing trauma as well as developing PTSD. Models that controlled for the twins' similarity of exposure to trauma found moderate heritabilities (30%–35%) for most of the individual symptoms, with nonshared environment explaining the rest of the variance in liability to developing PTSD, similar to the other anxiety disorders. Thus, genetic predisposition, when coupled with individual life experiences, moderates the likelihood of developing PTSD after a significant traumatic event. Although the majority of the traumatic events were likely combat-related, similar results obtained for a smaller subsample of 1,694 pairs who did not serve in Southeast Asia suggest that the VET Registry findings may generalize to civilian populations.

A second, smaller twin study extended these findings to female subjects with PTSD resulting from civilian traumas (Stein et al. 2002). The sample consisted of 291 female-female, 75 male-male, and 40 opposite-sex complete twin pairs ascertained from the general population in the Vancouver area of Canada. For pairs in which both twins were exposed to trauma, MZ pairs were more highly correlated than DZ pairs for all of the PTSD symptom clusters, and modeling results produced heritabilities for these clusters in a range similar to that found in the VET Registry study.

Molecular Genetic Studies

To this date, only dopaminergic system genes have been examined for association with PTSD. There is currently one positive and one negative report for association with the dopamine D_2 receptor. The dopamine transporter SLC6A3 VNTR polymorphism was examined in 102 chronic Israeli PTSD patients and 104 matched trauma survivors without PTSD. A significant excess of the 9-repeat allele was reported for the PTSD patients, suggesting (pending replication) that this polymorphism may increase vulnerability to developing PTSD in those who experience trauma (Segman et al. 2002).

Summary

Although PTSD is difficult to study with traditional genetic epidemiological methods, data from a few carefully crafted family and twin studies support a role for genetic factors in the development of PTSD, leading some research groups to begin the search for susceptibility genes for this condition.

Conclusion

A substantial volume of evidence exists to support the familial aggregation of all of the anxiety disorders. No significant differences emerge in the strength of this aggregation across disorders, with most ORs for rates of illness in first-degree relatives falling into the 4.0–6.0 range. Twin studies suggest that most, if not all, of this aggregation results from genetic effects, although the most evidence exists for PD. Molecular genetic studies of the ADs are still in their early stages, although again, the most evidence has thus far accumulated for PD.

Future studies will likely follow several directions. First, as in other complex medical illnesses, animal models can provide important advantages for studying psychiatric syndromes (Lander and Schork 1994). In particular, the face validity of animal models of fear compared with other psychiatric phenotypes (other than substance use syndromes) makes animal genetic studies an attractive starting point for identifying candidate anxiety susceptibility genes, and several groups have already begun to use this strategy.

Second, although the current classification of the anxiety disorders may have substantial clinical utility, it is unlikely that the biologic and genetic bases of these syndromes are as neatly delineated. The high rates of comorbidity among the ADs and with depressive disorders suggest shared risk factors which may include common susceptibility genes. However, the findings of family and twin studies regarding shared genetic vulnerability explaining the high rates of comorbidity of the ADs are, at face value, somewhat at odds with each other. Many, but not all, family studies observed had significantly increased rates of only the proband's disorder in relatives, especially when comorbidity in the proband was controlled for, suggesting relative specificity of familial risk. Twin studies found evidence for shared genetic risk across various ADs and with major depression. Several important differences may potentially account for some of these discrepancies, but discussion of these differences is outside of the scope of this review. If there are sources of genetic risk common to several syndromes, a more efficient and powerful strategy may be to identify candidate genes that increase risk across a range of disorders. When the data are examined across the diagnoses discussed in this chapter, there is accumulating evidence that several candidate genes may be associated with more than one disorder.

A third strategy is to replace clinical diagnoses by more basic, perhaps experimentally derived, phenotypes in molecular genetic analyses. There have been suggestions that clinical phenotypes measured by self-report may not reflect the underlying pathophysiological processes involved in the etiology of psychiatric disorders and, therefore, may not provide optimum targets for gene-finding strategies (Smoller and Tsuang 1998). Researchers interested in various psychiatric disorders have been attempting to identify potential endophenotypes that robustly reflect processes more proximal to gene expression involved in the development of psychopathology. One putative endophenotype already being explored is the increased sensitivity to panicogenic CO_2 inhalation in patients with panic disorder (Bellodi et al. 1998). Fear conditioning paradigms, if substantially correlated with clinical measures of anxiety, provide another potential endophenotype. Finally, personality measures such as neuroticism, which has been shown to increase risk across the internalizing disorders and to share genetic risk with major depression and GAD (Fanous et al. 2002; Hettema et al. 2004), may serve as semi-quantitative phenotypes in linkage and association studies.

References

Azzam A, Mathews CA: Meta-analysis of the association between the catecholamine-O-methyl-transferase gene and obsessive-compulsive disorder. Am J Med Genet B Neuropsychiatr Genet 123:64–69, 2003

Bellodi L, Sciuto G, Diaferia G, et al: Psychiatric disorders in the families of patients with obsessive-compulsive disorder. Psychiatry Res 42: 111–120, 1992

Bellodi L, Perna G, Caldirola D, et al: CO_2-induced panic attacks: a twin study. Am J Psychiatry 155:1184–1188, 1998

Billett EA, Richter MA, Sam F, et al: Investigation of dopamine system genes in obsessive-compulsive disorder. Psychiatr Genet 8:163–169, 1998

Black DW, Noyes R Jr, Goldstein RB, et al: A family study of obsessive-compulsive disorder. Arch Gen Psychiatry 49:362–368, 1992

Bradwejn J, Koszycki D, Shriqui C: Enhanced sensitivity to cholecystokinin tetrapeptide in panic disorder: clinical and behavioral findings. Arch Gen Psychiatry 48:603–610, 1991

Breslau N, Davis GC, Andreski P, et al: Traumatic events and posttraumatic stress disorder in an urban population of young adults. Arch Gen Psychiatry 48:216–222, 1991

Camarena B, Rinetti G, Cruz C, et al: Additional evidence that genetic variation of MAO-A gene supports a gender subtype in obsessive-compulsive disorder. Am J Med Genet 105:279–282, 2001

Carey G, Gottesman II: Twin and family studies of anxiety, phobic, and obsessive disorders, in Anxiety: New Research and Changing Concepts. Edited by Klein DF, Rabkin J. New York, Raven, 1981, pp 117–136

Clifford CA, Murray RM, Fulker DW: Genetic and environmental influences on obsessional traits and symptoms. Psychol Med 14:791–800, 1984

Crowe RR, Goedken R, Samuelson S, et al: Genomewide survey of panic disorder. Am J Med Genet 105:105–109, 2001

Deckert J, Nothen MM, Franke P, et al: Systematic mutation screening and association study of the A1 and A2a adenosine receptor genes in panic disorder suggest a contribution of the A2a gene to the development of disease. Mol Psychiatry 3:81–85, 1998

Fanous A, Gardner CO, Prescott CA, et al: Neuroticism, major depression and gender: a population-based twin study. Psychol Med 32: 719–728, 2002

Fyer AJ, Mannuzza S, Chapman TF, et al: A direct interview family study of social phobia. Arch Gen Psychiatry 50:286–293, 1993

Fyer AJ, Mannuzza S, Chapman TF, et al: Specificity in familial aggregation of phobic disorders. Arch Gen Psychiatry 52:564–573, 1995

Fyer AJ, Mannuzza S, Chapman TF, et al: Panic disorder and social phobia: effects of comorbidity on familial transmission. Anxiety 2:173–178, 1996

Gelernter J, Bonvicini K, Page G, et al: Linkage genome scan for loci predisposing to panic disorder or agoraphobia. Am J Med Genet 105: 548–557, 2001

Gelernter J, Page GP, Bonvicini K, et al: A chromosome 14 risk locus for simple phobia: results from a genomewide linkage scan. Mol Psychiatry 8:71–82, 2003

Gelernter J, Page GP, Stein MB, et al: Genome-wide linkage scan for loci predisposing to social phobia: evidence for a chromosome 16 risk locus. Am J Psychiatry 161:59–66, 2004

Goldstein RB, Wickramaratne PJ, Horwath E, et al: Familial aggregation and phenomenology of "early"-onset (at or before age 20 years) panic disorder. Arch Gen Psychiatry 54:271–278, 1997

Hamilton SP, Slager SL, Heiman GA, et al: Evidence for a susceptibility locus for panic disorder near the catechol-O-methyltransferase gene on chromosome 22. Biol Psychiatry 51:591–601, 2002

Hamilton SP, Fyer AJ, Durner M, et al: Further genetic evidence for a panic disorder syndrome mapping to chromosome 13q. Proc Natl Acad Sci USA 100:2550–2555, 2003

Hamilton SP, Slager SL, De Leon AB, et al: Evidence for genetic linkage between a polymorphism in the adenosine 2A receptor and panic disorder. Neuropsychopharmacology 29:558–565, 2004

Hanna GL, Veenstra-VanderWeele J, Cox NJ, et al: Genome-wide linkage analysis of families with obsessive-compulsive disorder ascertained through pediatric probands. Am J Med Genet 114:541–552, 2002

Hettema JM, Neale MC, Kendler KS: A review and meta-analysis of the genetic epidemiology of anxiety disorders. Am J Psychiatry 158:1568–1578, 2001a

Hettema JM, Prescott CA, Kendler KS: A population-based twin study of generalized anxiety disorder in men and women. J Nerv Ment Dis 189:413–420, 2001b

Hettema JM, Prescott CA, Kendler KS: Genetic and environmental sources of covariation between generalized anxiety disorder and neuroticism. Am J Psychiatry 161:1581–1587, 2004

Horwath E, Wolk SI, Goldstein RB, et al: Is the comorbidity between social phobia and panic disorder due to familial cotransmission or other factors? Arch Gen Psychiatry 52:574–582, 1995

Jonnal AH, Gardner CO, Prescott CA, et al: Obsessive and compulsive symptoms in a general population sample of female twins. Am J Med Genet 96:791–796, 2000

Karayiorgou M, Sobin C, Blundell ML, et al: Family-based association studies support a sexually dimorphic effect of COMT and MAOA on genetic susceptibility to obsessive-compulsive disorder. Biol Psychiatry 45:1178–1189, 1999

Kendler KS, Neale MC, Kessler RC, et al: Generalized anxiety disorder in women: a population based twin study. Arch Gen Psychiatry 49:267–272, 1992a

Kendler KS, Neale MC, Kessler RC, et al: The genetic epidemiology of phobias in women: the interrelationship of agoraphobia, social phobia, situational phobia, and simple phobia. Arch Gen Psychiatry 49: 273–281, 1992b

Kendler KS, Neale MC, Kessler RC, et al: Panic disorder in women: a population-based twin study. Psychol Med 23:397–406, 1993

Kendler KS, Gardner CO, Prescott CA: Panic syndromes in a population-based sample of male and female twins. Psychol Med 31:989–1000, 2001a

Kendler KS, Myers J, Prescott CA, et al: The genetic epidemiology of irrational fears and phobias in men. Arch Gen Psychiatry 58:257–265, 2001b

Kessler RC, McGonagle K, Zhao S, et al: Lifetime and 12-month prevalence of DSM-III-R psychiatric disorders in the United States: results from the National Comorbidity Survey. Arch Gen Psychiatry 51:8–19, 1994

Knowles JA, Fyer AJ, Vieland VJ, et al: Results of a genome-wide genetic screen for panic disorder. Am J Med Genet 81:139–147, 1998

Lander ES, Schork NJ: Genetic dissection of complex traits. Science 265: 2037–2048, 1994

Lesch KP, Bengel D, Heils A, et al: Association of anxiety-related traits with a polymorphism in the serotonin transporter gene regulatory region. Science 274:1527–1531, 1996

Logue MW, Vieland VJ, Goedken RJ, et al: Bayesian analysis of a previously published genome screen for panic disorder reveals new and compelling evidence for linkage to chromosome 7. Am J Med Genet B Neuropsychiatr Genet 121:95–99, 2003

Maier W, Lichtermann D, Minges J, et al: A controlled family study in panic disorder. J Psychiatr Res 27:79–87, 1993

Mannuzza S, Schneier FR, Chapman TF, et al: Generalized social phobia: reliability and validity. Arch Gen Psychiatry 52:230–237, 1995

Maser JD, Cloninger CR (eds): Comorbidity of Mood and Anxiety Disorders. Washington, DC, American Psychiatric Press, 1990

McKeon P, Murray R: Familial aspects of obsessive-compulsive neurosis. Br J Psychiatry 151:528–534, 1987

Mendlewicz J, Papadimitriou GN, Wilmotte J: Family study of panic disorder: comparison with generalized anxiety disorder, major depression and normal subjects. Psychiatr Genet 3:73–78, 1993

Neale MC, Walters EE, Eaves LJ, et al: Genetics of blood-injury fears and phobias: a population-based twin study. Am J Med Genet 54:326–334, 1994

Nestadt G, Samuels J, Riddle M, et al: A family study of obsessive-compulsive disorder. Arch Gen Psychiatry 57:358–363, 2000

Noyes R Jr, Hoehn-Saric R (eds): The Anxiety Disorders. Cambridge, England, Cambridge University Press, 1998

Noyes R Jr, Crowe RR, Harris E, et al: Relationship between panic disorder and agoraphobia: a family study. Arch Gen Psychiatry 43:227–232, 1986

Noyes R Jr, Clarkson C, Crowe RR, et al: A family study of generalized anxiety disorder. Am J Psychiatry 144:1019–1024, 1987

Pauls DL, Alsobrook JP, Goodman W, et al: A family study of obsessive-compulsive disorder. Am J Psychiatry 152:76–84, 1995

Rasmussen SA: Genetic studies of obsessive-compulsive disorder. Ann Clin Psychiatry 5:241–247, 1993

Rasmussen SA, Tsuang MT: Clinical characteristics and family history in DSM-III obsessive-compulsive disorder. Am J Psychiatry 143:317–322, 1986

Scherrer JF, True WR, Xian H, et al: Evidence for genetic influences common and specific to symptoms of generalized anxiety and panic. J Affect Disord 57:25–35, 2000

Segman RH, Cooper-Kazaz R, Macciardi F, et al: Association between the dopamine transporter gene and posttraumatic stress disorder. Mol Psychiatry 7:903–907, 2002

Skre I, Onstad S, Torgersen S, et al: A twin study of DSM-III-R anxiety disorders. Acta Psychiatr Scand 88:85–92, 1993

Smoller JW, Tsuang MT: Panic and phobic anxiety: defining phenotypes for genetic studies [see comments]. Am J Psychiatry 155:1152–1162, 1998

Stein MB, Chartier MJ, Hazen AL, et al: A direct-interview family study of generalized social phobia. Am J Psychiatry 155:90–97, 1998

Stein MB, Jang KL, Taylor S, et al: Genetic and environmental influences on trauma exposure and posttraumatic stress disorder symptoms: a twin study. Am J Psychiatry 159:1675–1681, 2002

Thorgeirsson TE, Oskarsson H, Desnica N, et al: Anxiety with panic disorder linked to chromosome 9q in Iceland. Am J Hum Genet 72:1221–1230, 2003

Torgersen S: The nature and origin of common phobic fears. Br J Psychiatry 134:343–351, 1979

True WR, Rice J, Eisen SA, et al: A twin study of genetic and environmental contributions to liability for posttraumatic stress symptoms. Arch Gen Psychiatry 50:257–264, 1993

Willour VL, Yao SY, Samuels J, et al: Replication study supports evidence for linkage to 9p24 in obsessive-compulsive disorder. Am J Hum Genet 75:508–513, 2004

Woo JM, Yoon KS, Yu BH: Catechol O-methyltransferase genetic polymorphism in panic disorder. Am J Psychiatry 159:1785–1787, 2002

Yamada K, Hattori E, Shimizu M, et al: Association studies of the cholecystokinin B receptor and A2a adenosine receptor genes in panic disorder. J Neural Transm 108:837–848, 2001

Zhang H, Leckman JF, Pauls DL, et al: Genomewide scan of hoarding in sib pairs in which both sibs have Gilles de la Tourette syndrome. Am J Hum Genet 70:896–904, 2002

Chapter 5

Genetics of Substance Use Disorders

Carol A. Prescott, Ph.D.
Hermine H. Maes, Ph.D.
Kenneth S. Kendler, M.D.

Substance use disorders (SUDs) have an enormous societal cost. In addition to the physical and psychological disability experienced by those who are addicted, the costs to society include crime, accidents, an overburdened judicial system, lost earnings, and disrupted families and social relations (Room et al. 2003). The economic impact of substance abuse in the United States is estimated to exceed a cost of $420 billion annually (Rice 1999).

Recent years have seen increased public recognition and media attention to the seriousness of SUDs, and more individuals are seeking treatment. However, treatment availability lags far behind need. Among those seeking treatment, a majority are likely to experience relapse. The early onset of SUDs means that affected individuals may not successfully accomplish the important social and occupational developmental tasks associated with adolescence and early adulthood. The chronicity and poor treatment outcomes indicate years of impairment or episodes of impairment that may seriously disrupt functioning. These aspects underscore the importance of prevention and the need for treatments that prevent relapse. Research addressing genetic influences on SUDs has contributed to a better understanding of etiology, which is expected to improve prevention and intervention efforts.

In this chapter, we discuss why genetic research on SUDs was begun and consider some aspects of addictions research that differ from research on other psychiatric disorders. We then review the results from genetic epidemiological studies and molecular genetic studies from each of three groups of substances: alcohol, nicotine, and illicit substances. Finally, we discuss the implications of these findings for understanding the development of SUDs and look ahead to where future research may lead.

We note that our literature review is not comprehensive; a detailed review of all the literature on these topics is beyond the scope of a single chapter. We have confined our review to studies of humans, although much animal work is being conducted that may assist in identifying genes influencing aspects of addictions. We have taken the strategy of presenting results from major studies that employed standardized assessment methods (usually diagnostic interviews) and had sample sizes adequate for drawing meaningful conclusions about genetic effects. We have also focused on studies of adults, for whom knowledge about SUD outcomes is more complete. For studies that have generated multiple papers and findings, we have attempted to cite recent reports that can be used to find earlier work. Details of many studies summarized here can be found in the review chapter by Ball and Collier (2002).

Rationale for the Study of Genetic Influences on Substance Use and Abuse

Although the biological basis for psychiatric disorders has gained widespread public acceptance, this gain has not necessarily been extended to SUDs. Many professionals and laypersons are reluctant to apply the label of "illness" to behaviors that are viewed as arising from poor self-control or deprived environments. Consequently, some readers may wonder why genetic studies have been conducted on SUDs.

Until recently most genetic research on addictions has focused on alcoholism, so we begin our discussion with this SUD. Three lines of evidence from alcohol research suggested that genetic studies of alcoholism were a potentially fruitful endeavor:

First, animal breeding studies, primarily with rodents, found that a wide range of alcohol-related behaviors appeared to have a genetic basis. For example, rats were selectively bred for their preference to drink an alcohol solution versus water without alcohol. After several generations, there was virtually no overlap in the two groups: rats who preferred alcohol produced pups that preferred alcohol—strong evidence that variation in behavior was due to genetic factors.

Second, it has long been recognized that alcoholism runs in families. In a review based on more than 50 studies, Cotton (1979) concluded that individuals with a first-degree alcoholic relative have a two- to fourfold increased risk for alcoholism compared with individuals without a family history. Although this association could be due to environmental factors shared by family members, it could also be due to transmission of genes between generations.

Third, ethnic variation in liver enzymes involved in the metabolism of alcohol is related to differences in risk for alcoholism. Individuals from some Asian groups have a high frequency of the low-activity allele of the aldehyde dehydrogenase gene (*ALDH2*). This allele is associated with slower catalysis of acetaldehyde into acetic acid, which results in a buildup, after alcohol consumption, of acetaldehyde, producing facial flushing, nausea, and other unpleasant effects. Individuals homozygous for this allele are at very low risk for developing alcoholism because of their inability to metabolize even small amounts of ethanol.

Challenges in Research on the Genetics of Addictions

As described in Chapter 2 ("Questions, Models, and Methods in Psychiatric Genetics"), several challenges confront researchers conducting research in genetic epidemiology. As with other psychiatric disorders, the issues of phenotype definition and measurement pertain to addictions. However, substance abuse research has additional complications not encountered (or encountered to a lesser extent) when studying other psychiatric disorders. We discuss these issues briefly here because they influence our ability to summarize the relevant literature in this field.

One important issue is that studies of SUDs are difficult to compare across cultures or historical periods. Societal interventions, such as prohibition in the United States in the early 20th century, or the more recent opening of borders in Eastern Europe, produced rapid changes in the availability of psychoactive substances. Changing social norms about the acceptability of drugs influence the probability of use and also affect individuals' willingness to disclose their use and related symptoms.

The prevalences of use and abuse of illicit substances vary widely even across regions of the United States within the same period. Furthermore, studies of family members from different generations are complicated by the varying availability of drugs during the periods when individuals were at greatest risk to initiate substance use.

Most psychiatric disorders are assumed to be multifactorial in origin, arising from a combination of genetic and environmental risk factors. For the other disorders reviewed in this book, environmental risk is ubiquitous; although the level of stress varies, no one has a stress-free life. For SUDs, however, major (and necessary) risk factors are the availability and sufficient consumption of the substance. Exposure to this risk factor is not universal, is to some degree self-initiated, and is probably not random with respect to genetic risk. Among individuals who have a family history of substance abuse (and thus have above-average genetic risk), some will have increased environmental risk (the substance is used by members of their household), and others will have decreased environmental risk (associated with a repugnance for substance use arising from witnessing its adverse effects in relatives).

Finally, as described in more detail subsequently, the processes that determine exposure to a substance are likely to differ from those that affect development of addiction once drug exposure has occurred. Some evidence suggests that environmental factors shared by family members are important for exposure but are less important for the development of dependence contingent on exposure.

Alcoholism

Research on genetic influences on the etiology of alcoholism can be organized into two major categories. *Genetic epidemiological designs* use the prevalence and concordance of disorders among individuals with varying genetic and environmental similarity to infer the role of genetic factors. *Molecular genetic studies* assess genetic influence explicitly by measuring genetic variation and its association with a disorder. More details about these approaches are presented in Chapter 1 ("Introduction") and Chapter 2.

Genetic Epidemiological Studies

The two major types of designs used in genetic epidemiology are *adoption studies* and *twin studies* (see Chapter 2). The conceptual model used in the adoption and twin studies reviewed here assumes that multiple genetic and environmental factors combine to increase or decrease an individual's vulnerability to develop an SUD. This vulnerability is assumed to be continuous and normally distributed, even though for research purposes individuals are usually divided into two categories: affected or not.

Adoption Studies

Adoption studies permit estimation of the separate effects of genetic factors and rearing environment because adoptees receive their genes from one set of parents and family environment from another set. Two assumptions of the adoption design are that the effects of the intrauterine environment are negligible and the choice of adoptive family is random with respect to risk factors for alcoholism (i.e., no selective placement). Under these conditions, the degree to which adoptees resemble their adoptive relatives is a direct measure of the influence of family environment and the degree to which they resemble their biological relatives is a measure of genetic influence.

There have been five adoption studies of alcoholism in females and six in males that contained adequate sample sizes (Figure 5–1). (An early study conducted by Roe and Burks [1945] is historically noteworthy but included only 36 individuals with a family history positive for alcoholism, too few to draw meaningful inferences.) One study conducted in Denmark (Goodwin et al. 1973) and two conducted in metropolitan areas of Sweden (Stockholm and Gothenburg; Cloninger et al. 1981; Sigvardsson et al. 1996) matched government birth registries against temperance

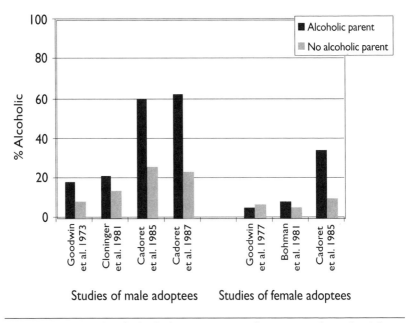

Figure 5–1. Risk of alcoholism among adoptees with and without biological alcoholic parents.

board registration (TBR) records of alcoholism treatment or alcohol-related offenses. This approach enabled the researchers to identify adults who had been adopted and determine whether their biological parents had a history of alcohol abuse. Two other studies were conducted with samples of adoptees identified from public and private adoption records in the state of Iowa (e.g., Cadoret et al. 1987; Langbehn et al. 2003). The biological parents in the Iowa studies were classified into those with and without alcohol problems on the basis of interviews with biological mothers conducted at the time of the adoption. Adoptees in all these studies were classified as "family history negative" if neither parent had evidence of alcoholism, and as "family history positive" if at least one biological parent had evidence of alcoholism. The status of the adoptees was determined in adulthood from personal psychiatric evaluations and public records.

All five studies of male adoptees found evidence for genetic contributions to risk for alcoholism. Adopted men with a positive family history were at significantly higher risk for alcoholism, with increased risk ranging from 1.6 to 3.6 times that of males with a negative family history. The studies of female adoptees obtained mixed results, with two supporting genetic influences and two finding no evidence of genetic transmission. The studies based on samples collected in Stockholm (Bohman et al. 1981) and Iowa found significantly increased risk of alcoholism among women adopted away from alcoholic parents compared with women with a negative family history, with risk ratios of 1.6 and 6.3, respectively. However, the studies conducted in Gothenburg (Sigvardsson et al. 1996) and Denmark (Goodwin et al. 1977) found no significant differences between the groups.

In all these studies, most parents were not formally evaluated, so the parental diagnoses are imprecise. It is also likely that alcoholism went undetected in some biological parents. The effects of this underdiagnosis would be to reduce the difference between the family history positive and negative cases, making it less likely to detect genetic influences. Thus, the consistency observed across studies of male adoptees is all the more impressive. This work had a substantial impact on altering perspectives among researchers and mental health professionals about the possibility of genetic influences on SUDs.

Twin Studies

Estimates of genetic and environmental contributions to risk for a disorder are obtained from twin studies by comparing the resemblance of identical (monozygotic, or MZ) and fraternal (dizygotic, or DZ) twin pairs. To the degree that pair resemblance among MZ pairs exceeds that of DZ pairs, genetic factors are implicated in vulnerability to addiction. If MZ and DZ pairs are equally similar, this indicates that shared environmental factors are contributing to variation in risk. To the extent that members of MZ pairs are dissimilar, this implicates the role of individual specific environmental sources. Given certain assumptions (see Chapters 1 and 2), population variation in vulnerability can be partitioned into three sources: 1) genetic variation comes from genes whose allelic effects combine additively; 2) family or common environment includes all environmental factors that make relatives more similar; and 3) individual-specific environment includes all remaining factors not shared by family members.

There have been 10 major twin studies of alcoholism, and the results have varied with the method used to identify participants (Figure 5–2; see Prescott 2001). Three studies identified affected individuals (probands) through treatment settings or archival records and then assessed the clinical status of their co-twins through individual follow-up. All three studies obtained evidence for significant genetic influences on alcoholism in men, with heritability estimates ranging from 36% to 70% (Kaij 1960; McGue et al. 1992; Prescott et al. 2005). In the three studies that included women, the evidence for genetic influences was weaker, with heritability estimates ranging from 0% to 26%. However, because of the smaller numbers of female pairs, these results are limited by low power. Twin studies using proband ascertainment are the only ones that have found consistent evidence for environmental factors contributing to familial similarity for alcoholism. Estimates of common environmental variance were 10%–51% in males and 29%–67% in females.

Another four studies matched twin registries against archival information (including TBR, military and medical records) to classify pairs into those in which both twins had data suggesting alcoholism, those with only one twin identified, and those with neither twin identified. Two of the four studies included female twins, but the prevalence of alcoholism in women was less than 1%, resulting in very low power to obtain accurate estimates. In these studies, the case identification method and low prevalences of alcoholism suggest the samples were selected for severe cases. Alcoholic co-twins who had not been hospitalized or identified by TBR would have gone undetected, leading to underestimates of how many pairs were similar for alcoholism. Given these limitations, the estimates obtained with this design are fairly similar, with heritability estimates among males of 32%–59% and common environmental effects of 0%–25%. The one study containing an adequate number of female twin pairs was based on hospitalization records from Sweden. Analyses based on this sample initially reported low heritability, but a recent follow-up of this sample

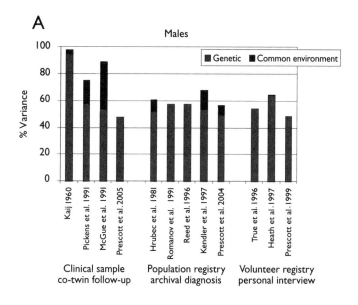

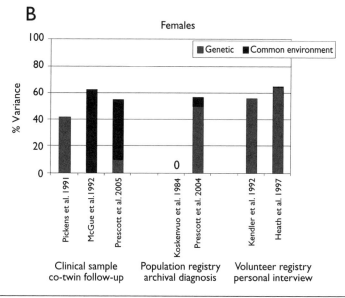

Figure 5–2. Genetic and environmental proportions of variance in alcoholism estimated from studies of adult twins.

0 = heritability estimate of 0%.

See Prescott 2001 for citations of original studies. When studies reported estimates for multiple definitions, results based on narrow definitions were used.

resulted in an upward revision of these estimates (J.W. Kuhn, N.L. Pedersen, unpublished data, 2004). The other three twin studies of alcoholism used population-based twin registries: our own study, the Virginia Adult Twin Study of Psychiatric and Substance Use Disorders (VATSPSUD; Prescott et al. 1999); the Vietnam Era Twin Study (VETS; True et al. 1996); and a national twin registry from Australia (Heath et al. 1997). Participants were unselected for alcoholism, and all were assessed by personal interview for history of alcoholism. The results of these studies are quite consistent. All three studies of males and the two that included females found heritability estimates of 55%–65% and negligible (<10%) estimates of common environmental effects.

In summary, the results of twin studies of males have consistently found resemblance among MZ twin pairs to be significantly greater than among DZ pairs, implicating a significant role for genetic factors in contributing to vulnerability to develop alcoholism. The heritability estimates in most studies suggest that genetic variability accounts for 50%–60% of the variation in risk for alcoholism. In contrast, studies of female twins are less consistent. Those based on samples identified through treatment settings suggested familiality of alcoholism among women is due to shared environments rather than to genetic factors, whereas studies using population-based twin registries found genetic influences on alcoholism to be of similar magnitude in males and females. Our interpretation is that these differences are more likely to be methodological (based on procedural differences between types of studies) than substantive, but a final resolution may require the identification of specific genes and biological mechanisms.

Molecular Genetic Studies

The goal of measured gene studies is to identify *susceptibility loci*, regions of the genome that contain genes that increase or decrease risk for developing a disorder. The most commonly used design is the case-control association study that compares the frequency of candidate gene alleles in groups of individuals with and without alcoholism. Within-family association designs test whether particular alleles are more likely to be shared by family members who have the same disease status (having alcoholism or not) than by those who differ in status. Genetic linkage studies take a complementary approach, searching for regions of the genome that are shared by family members who have alcoholism (i.e., "linked") and then identifying the genes that are located in those regions.

Association Studies

Association studies of alcoholism are quite recent, but the literature has accumulated rapidly. The possible candidates include virtually any gene expressed in the brain, as well as those involved in alcohol metabolism. The extensiveness and rapidly changing nature of the literature make it difficult to offer a concise summary of association findings. We focus our discussion on candidate genes that have been associated with alcoholism in human studies and that have been verified in at least one independent replication study. There is also a large literature on candidate genes arising from animal studies of alcohol-related behaviors, such as sensitivity, tolerance, sedation, and withdrawal. These genes are of potential relevance to understanding the etiology of alcoholism but are beyond the scope of this chapter (for review, see Crabbe 2002).

Obvious candidates for susceptibility loci are genes that influence variation in the metabolism of ethanol. The most commonly studied is *ALDH*, described above, which has strong protective effects in some Asian populations but does not account for much of the risk in other ethnic groups. However, there are other genes with greater variability in non-Asian groups that code for enzymes affecting alcohol metabolism, including several alcohol dehydrogenase (ADH) and cytochrome P450 variants.

Association studies of alcoholism based on neurotransmitter systems began in 1991 with a publication by Blum and colleagues (1991) of increased risk for alcoholism associated with the AI allele near the region coding for the dopamine D_2 receptor (*DRD2*). This was followed by a series of replication attempts, most of which did not confirm this association. Subsequently, positive associations have been found for many other candidates, including the dopamine D_4 receptor (*DRD4*), the dopamine transporter (*DAT*), neuropeptide Y (*NPY*), monoamine oxidase (*MAO*), the GABA system, and others. The finding that opiate antagonists (i.e., substances that interfere with opiate receptor activity) are also effective for preventing craving in alcoholism has sparked interest in opiate systems. A focus of much recent interest is the serotonin transporter promoter (*5HTTLPR*). At least six independent studies have found the short variant to be associated with increased risk for alcoholism or violent/antisocial alcoholism. However, in all these systems, there are negative as well as positive reports of association with alcoholism, so this field must be considered in an early phase. A detailed description of results from human association studies is given in Dick and Foroud (2003).

Linkage Studies

Several linkage studies of alcoholism have been conducted, and more are under way. The largest of these studies, the Collaborative Study on the Genetics of Alcoholism (COGA; see, e.g., Foroud et al. 2000), includes three different samples of multiplex pedigrees (extended families with multiple individuals affected) with alcoholism collected throughout the United States. The data from the first two samples, consisting of 262 families, have been analyzed and have yielded some promising findings, including evidence for susceptibility loci on chromosomes 1, 2, 4, 5, 7, and 15. Linkage data from the first COGA sample were provided to investigators participating in the 11th Genetic Analysis Workshop and resulted in identification of other regions of interest (Saccone et al. 2003). A noteworthy feature of this study is the availability of alternative phenotypes (including subjective response to ethanol, drinking quantity, electrophysiological response, and psychometrically defined phenotypes) and investigation of the role of alcoholism subtypes and comorbidity patterns. For example, the evidence for linkage to the chromosome 1 region was strengthened with the use of a broad definition of affected status, which included depression with or without alcoholism (Nurnberger et al. 2001).

Long and colleagues (1998) studied a sample of 152 individuals from 32 multiplex pedigrees from a Southwestern American Indian tribe selected for having very high prevalence of alcoholism. Among other findings, results from this study strongly support the existence of susceptibility loci on chromosome 4 in a region containing the *ADH* cluster.

Results from a genome scan based on 330 individuals from 65 multiplex families ascertained in the Pittsburgh area were reported by Hill and colleagues (2004). These others found evidence for linkage to alcoholism on chromosomes 6, 7, and 17 (based on LOD scores > 3.0). Including age, sex, personality, and electrophysiological measures as covariates increased the evidence for linkage in these areas and identified several other regions of interest close to regions that had also been identified in reports based on the COGA study.

A fourth study, by Ehlers and colleagues (2004) was based on a genome scan of 245 individuals from 41 families recruited from Mission Indian reservations. Initial results from this study include weak evidence for linkage (LOD > 2.0) to alcoholism severity on chromosomes 4 and 12 and to alcoholism withdrawal on chromosomes 6, 15, and 16.

In summary, the available linkage results for alcoholism are promising, and follow-up analyses are yielding evidence for particular genes. There is consistent evidence from three published studies (Foroud et al. 2000; Long et al. 1998; Ehlers et al. 2004) for involvement of a region of chromosome 4 near the *ADH* cluster. In addition, initial results from our study of 511 affected sibling pairs collected in Ireland indicate strong linkage of severity of alcohol dependence to this region (Prescott et al., in press).

Smoking and Nicotine Dependence

Genetic Epidemiological Studies

Relatively few twin and adoption studies have been conducted that used nicotine dependence as an outcome. More commonly, twin studies have used measures such as number of cigarettes consumed or persistence of smoking, which serve as rough proxies for nicotine dependence. We therefore review studies of nicotine use as well as of nicotine dependence.

Twin Studies

We summarize studies that have examined *lifetime* or current use of tobacco products (which we will term *smoking initiation*) and those that have examined actual nicotine dependence or its proxies. There are more than 15 published twin studies of smoking initiation among adults, originating from seven different countries. Detailed reviews of this literature have been published by Sullivan and Kendler (1997), Heath et al. (1998), and Li (2003). Estimates of the heritability of smoking initiation were generally high, with most values falling between 40% and 70% (median= 57%). Estimates of the proportion of variance in liability due to shared environmental effects were more variable, with most ranging from 0% to 50%. The median estimate for the contribution of individual-specific environmental effects was 25%. One of the most striking aspects of this literature is the consistent evidence for moderate to high heritability estimates for a wide range of ages and countries and for both genders (Madden et al. 2004).

There have been eight reported twin studies based on nicotine dependence or its proxies that permit calculation of heritability estimates (Figure 5–3). These results are based on 17 samples collected in the United States, Australia, Sweden, and Finland. The most common phenotype examined is *persistence,* which is defined only among individuals who have ever smoked and which distinguishes between those who are a current versus an ex-smoker. Median estimates across these studies are as follows: heritability, 54%; common environment, 12%; and specific environment, 35%. It is noteworthy that heritability estimates tend to be higher for the two studies that use direct measures of nicotine dependence.

Adoption Studies

Five studies have examined smoking initiation in twins reared apart, a combination of the twin and adoption study designs. Concordance for smoking in the 147 MZ twin pairs reported in these studies was high (75%) and only slightly lower than the concordance rate reported from studies of MZ twins reared together (84%) (see Sullivan and Kendler 1997; Kendler et al. 2000).

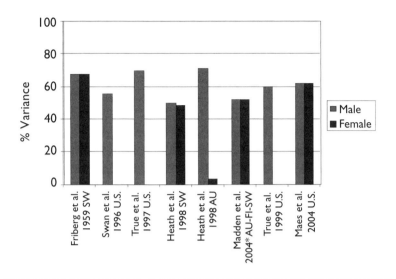

Figure 5–3. Genetic contributions to smoking persistence or nicotine dependence estimated from studies of adult twins.
AU = Australia, FI = Finland, SW = Sweden, U.S. = United States. Studies by Swan (1998) and True (1997, 1999) were based on male twins only.
*Median of age groups and samples.
See Maes et al. 2004 for citations of original studies.

The two available adoption studies reported substantial correlations for smoking status between biological parents and offspring, but not between adoptive parents and their adoptive offspring. Similarly, correlations between biological siblings (either non-twin siblings or DZ twins) were significantly different from zero, while those between adoptive siblings were not. In aggregate, the reared-apart twin studies and adoption studies confirm the hypothesis of strong genetic influences on smoking initiation and nicotine dependence.

Molecular Genetic Studies

In contrast to the extensive literature on genetic epidemiological studies of smoking behavior and nicotine dependence, gene-finding approaches have been fewer but are becoming more common, reflecting the general trend in the genetic analysis of complex traits.

Linkage Studies

Genome scans of smoking-related measures have been completed by four different research groups, and others are under way in the United Kingdom, Australia, and Finland. The first was conducted with two samples of sibling pairs concordant for nicotine dependence, one from Christchurch, New Zealand, and a second from Richmond, Virginia (Straub et al. 1999). A genome scan of 451 markers on the New Zealand sample produced modest evidence for linkage on chromosome 2 and weaker linkage signals on chromosomes 4, 10, 16, 17, and 18. Weak evidence for replication with the independent Richmond sample was observed on chromosomes 2, 16, and 17.

Several studies based on data from the COGA study have examined linkage for smoking-related traits, including smoking initiation, "pack-years," and "habitual smoking" (e.g., Bierut et al. 2004). Relatively strong evidence for linkage of pack-years was observed for chromosome 5q. Modest evidence for linkage was found for regions on chromosomes 2, 3, 4, 6, 9, 11, 14, 15, 17, and 21, but with few replications across reports.

Data from a 400-marker genome scan with 330 extended families participating in the Framingham Heart Study were made available to investigators participating in the 13th Genetic Analysis Workshop, resulting in several reports (Saccone et al. 2003). The strongest evidence for linkage to smoking status was reported for chromosomes 11 and 20, with suggestive linkage to chromosomes 2, 4, 5, 7, 9, 13, 14, 17, and 22.

As part of a U.S.-Dutch collaborative project on the genetics of smoking initiation and nicotine dependence, a 379-marker genome scan was performed on 646 sibling pairs for the two phenotypes of smoking initiation and number of cigarettes smoked. Suggestive linkage was found on chromosomes 6, 10, and 14 for smoking initiation and on chromosomes 3 and 10 for number of cigarettes smoked (Vink et al. 2004).

Most linkage studies of nicotine dependence are relatively recent or still in progress, and thus cross-study comparisons are difficult to make. Although several chromosomes are implicated in more than one sample, they do not necessarily imply replications, as the regions may not overlap. Furthermore, because of multiple testing, there is the possibility that the results include false positives. We look forward to resolution of these issues through future collaborations and meta-analyses.

Association Studies

The growing number of association studies of candidate genes for smoking initiation and nicotine dependence are described in recent reviews (Batra et al. 2003; Lerman and Berrettini 2003). In summary, they can be divided into four broad categories related to the metabolism of nicotine, nicotine receptors, the dopaminergic system, and the serotonergic system.

First, genes in the cytochrome P450 system that influence the metabolism of nicotine constitute obvious candidates. Interest has focused on the genes for CYP2A6 and CYP2D6, both of which are involved in the metabolism of nicotine to cotinine and have low activity variants. Results have been contradictory, with some studies showing an association with smoking behavior and others not showing such an association.

A second possible group of candidates are genes involved in sensitivity to nicotine, the major addictive substance in tobacco. Evidence from mouse knockouts suggests that the gene coding for the nicotinic acetylcholine receptor β_2 subunit (CHRNB2) is necessary for the full reinforcing properties of nicotine. However, studies of humans have not yet identified any variations in CHRNB2 associated with substance initiation or nicotine dependence. Some evidence suggests variation in CHRNA4 may be associated with reduced risk for nicotine addiction.

A third group of possible candidates comprise genes involved in the dopaminergic system, which have been examined in association with smoking. This avenue of research was motivated by findings suggesting that the mesolimbic dopaminergic system appears to play a significant role in the reinforcing effects of addictive drugs, including nicotine. A number of studies have examined the association between several aspects of smoking behavior and variants in the dopamine receptor genes DRD1, DRD2, and DRD4 and a repeat polymorphism in the dopamine transporter protein gene (DAT). Findings have been fairly typical in that initial strongly positive results could not be replicated in more recent, and probably more carefully performed, studies. A small number of studies have examined genes related to dopamine synthesis or degradation, including those for monoamine oxidase–B (MAO-B), monoamine oxidase–A (MAO-A), dopamine ß-hydroxylase, and catechol-*O*-methyltransferase (COMT), with mixed results. Several studies examining polymorphisms in the tyrosine hydroxylase gene among smokers initially obtained negative results, but they did replicate associations between tobacco use and the *K4* allele of the tyrosine hydroxylase gene.

The fourth group of possible candidate genes examined in association studies of smoking involves the serotonergic system, based on evidence that nicotine withdrawal may be modulated by serotonergic transmission. The most-studied gene in this system is that for the serotonin transporter (5-HTT), particularly the functional polymorphism also implicated in alcoholism and major depression (*5HTTLPR*). To date these studies have produced conflicting results. Variation in another serotonergic system gene, the tryptophan hydroxylase gene, has been associated with age at onset of smoking.

In summary, this area of research is in an early stage and may be limited by several methodological weaknesses. Most studies have not examined nicotine dependence directly but have used current smoking status as the outcome. Sample sizes have tended to be relatively modest, and the statistical criteria have tended to be liberal, perhaps leading to false positive results.

Abuse of and Dependence on Illicit Substances

Genetic Epidemiological Studies

Few genetic epidemiological studies have been conducted on illicit drugs, in part because of the relatively short history of research on addictive substances other than alcohol and tobacco. Because of secular changes in drug availability across generations, most studies have been conducted among individuals in the same generation (such as twins) or have examined the relationship between alcoholism in the parental generation and drug use in their offspring.

Family and Adoption Studies

Relatives of individuals with addictions to illicit drugs have been found to be at increased risk for a range of other disorders, including addiction to other drugs, alcoholism, depression, and antisocial personality disorder (e.g., Merikangas et al. 1998). Results from the adoption study by Cadoret and colleagues in Iowa suggest that these associations are due to genetic factors (Langbehn et al. 2003) and also underscore the complexity of the etiology of SUDs. Drug abuse in male adoptees was significantly associated with alcoholism, drug abuse, and antisocial personality in biological parents. In addition, psychiatric disorders among adoptive parents increased risk for adoptee antisocial personality, which was then associated with higher prevalence of drug abuse.

Twin Studies

There have been three studies of illicit drug abuse that involved adult twins assessed with clinical interviews and that reported heritability values separately by class of substance. (Another small study by Gynther et al. [1995] reported twin pair resemblance for illicit substances combined across drug class.) Two were based on population twin registries (VETS, Tsuang et al. 1996, 1998; VATSPSUD, see citations in Kendler et al. 1999a), and the other identified participants through treatment settings in Minnesota (van den Bree et al. 1998). For cannabis, sedatives, stimulants, cocaine, hallucinogens, and opiates, the evidence suggests that genetic factors account for a substantial proportion of the population variation in risk for development of drug abuse and dependence. The estimated heritabilities range from 25% to 79%, with most being in the range of 55% to 75% (Figure 5–4). Although estimates vary across sexes and substances, in most cases they are not significantly different, in part due to the relatively low prevalences of most SUDs.

Molecular Genetic Studies

The candidate genes tested for illicit drugs are similar to those described for alcohol and nicotine, including genes involved in the reward system, as well as those for receptors for specific drug

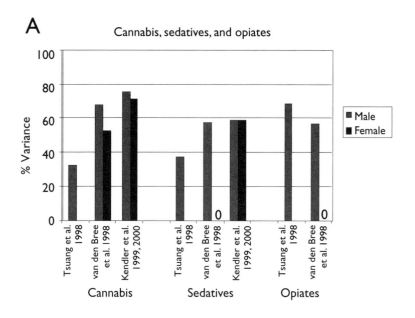

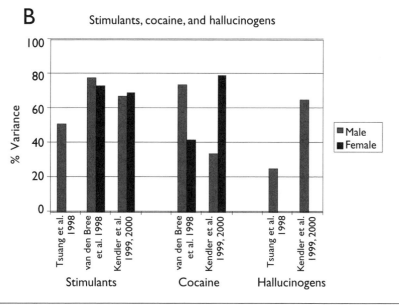

Figure 5–4. Genetic contributions to illict drug abuse/dependence estimated from studies of adult twins.

0 = heritability estimate of 0%.

See Ball and Collier 2002 for citations of original studies.

classes. Many studies are under way, but thus far few findings have been replicated, and most of the genes involved are not known to have functions related to the actions of the drug class studied (e.g., Kreek et al. 2004). Positive findings have been reported for variants in several systems, including the dopamine$_2$ (*DRD2*) and μ opiate receptor genes. Data collection for several linkage studies for illicit drugs is under way, but as of this writing, few results are available.

Influence of Genetic Variation on Risk for Substance Use Disorders

Research pertaining to genetic influences on the etiology of SUDs occurs at many levels of analysis, from the molecular to the familial. Figure 5–5 portrays some of the ways susceptibility loci are hypothesized to influence risk for SUDs. This schematic diagram not only portrays the complexity of SUD etiology but also underscores the lack of current knowledge about specific mechanisms and connections between levels of analysis. In this section, we describe several approaches being used to understand the mechanisms underlying genetic influences on substance use disorders.

Genetic Influences on Stages of Substance Use

Recent work in the genetic epidemiology of SUDs is investigating whether the stages of substance use differ in their genetic and environmental origins. For example, the influences on initiation of substance use may be predominantly environmental (e.g., peers, cultural factors), whereas risk for developing dependence once substance use has begun may be attributable more to genetic factors (e.g., influencing physiological and pharmacological response). Failure to account for different origins in substance use stages may lead to erroneous estimates from twin studies, particularly if a large proportion of the population never initiates substance use. If individuals who are genetically vulnerable to develop dependence never try the substance, they will not express their risk, leading to underestimates of genetic influences on the development of dependence from twin studies. This po-

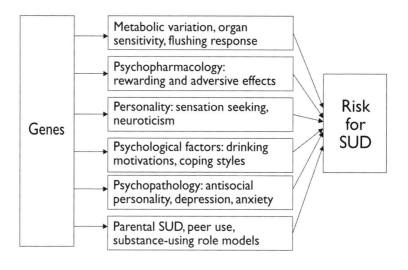

Figure 5–5.   Schematic representation of the pathways by which genes influence risk for substance use disorders.

tential source of underestimation is less of a concern in studies of alcohol, where exposure is nearly universal in Western samples, but is an important consideration when interpreting results from studies of other substance use disorders.

Figure 5–6 portrays a twin model developed by Michael Neale and Kenneth Kendler to estimate the genetic and environmental influences on substance dependence conditional upon initiation of substance use (e.g., Kendler et al. 1999b). The influences on dependence arise in part from the factors underlying initiation and in part from those factors specific to substance dependence. This model was first applied to smoking initiation and nicotine dependence in adult female twins from the VATSPSUD and has been applied to tobacco data in three other studies, including the only nationally representative twin plus sibling pair sample available from the United States (*N*=2,916 individuals, ascertained under the auspices of the MacArthur Foundation; K.S. Kendler, K.C. Jacobson, M.C. Neale, et al., unpublished data, 2000). This study concluded that the genetic risk factors for heavy smoking (estimated heritability of 72%) were about equally divided between those specific to heavy smoking and those shared with smoking initiation. An expanded three-stage model that included initiation, regular use, and dependence has recently been applied to data from the VATSPSUD (Maes et al. 2004). This study found that the genetic effects on nicotine dependence could be about equally divided into those shared with smoking initiation and regular use, those shared with regular use alone, and those uniquely affecting progression to nicotine dependence. The linkage of both the smoking initiation and number of cigarettes phenotypes to the same region of chromosome 10 (Vink et al. 2004) provides further evidence of shared genetic vulnerability to initiation and dependence.

The two-stage model (Figure 5–6) has also been applied to data on use of illicit substances among female twins from the VATSPSUD (Kendler et al. 1999a). The results differed somewhat across substances, but two major findings are noteworthy. There were genetic factors that specifically affect the risk for progression from use to abuse or dependence. Second, although environmental factors shared by twins were an important influence on the stage of drug initiation, there was no evidence that they affected the development of abuse or dependence beyond their influence on initiation.

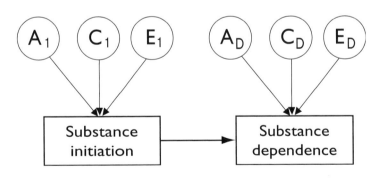

Figure 5–6. Contingent causal pathway model for the development of substance dependence.
A = additive genetic effects; C = common environmental effects; E = individual specific environmental effects.

Specificity of Genetic Effects

Another important issue is whether genes affecting SUDs are substance-specific or confer a more general predisposition to developing other forms of SUD and psychopathology. In U.S. epidemiological studies, more than 50% of individuals who meet the diagnostic criteria for an addictive disorder have at least one other disorder (Kessler et al. 1997). Most often these are another addictive disorder, depression, anxiety, or antisocial personality.

Several family studies of multiple substances have concluded that risk is not specific to a drug class (Merikangas et al. 1998). For example, relatives of smokers have higher risk for alcoholism and SUD than do relatives of nonsmokers. A few studies have found evidence of familiality for specific drugs classes, including cocaine and cannabis. However, this effect could be due to genetic factors shared by family members or to cultural or familial influence on drug availability and preference.

The specificity question can be better resolved by means of twin studies of the overlap across drug categories. If addiction to a substance in one twin is associated with higher than chance levels of addiction to another substance in the co-twin, and the rates of cross-substance, cross-twin addiction are higher in MZ than DZ pairs, this provides evidence for the existence of general genetic factors for addiction. All five studies that have used this approach with adult twins found significant genetic overlap for smoking with alcoholism or heavy drinking. Two twin studies reported on the overlap across classes of illicit drugs and found that a single genetic factor contributed to risk for addiction to all classes of drugs. In the VETS study, the specific genetic effects varied across substance classes but were particularly important for opiate addiction (Tsuang et al. 1998). In analyses of data from the VATSPSUD study, there was strong evidence for common genetic influences and little evidence for substance-specific genetic effects (e.g., Kendler et al. 2003a).

Molecular genetic strategies have also provided evidence relevant to the specificity-generality issue. Uhl et al. (2002) attempted to map susceptibility loci that influence abuse of a broad range of substances. The available results from association studies suggest that candidate genes have diverse effects and may influence risk for dependence on a variety of substances and through multiple mechanisms. These results are consistent with the existence of genetic factors that mediate variation in the reward system or through personality variation.

Genetic Influences on Substance Use Disorders: Psychopathology Comorbidity

A related issue to genetic specificity is the degree to which shared genes can explain the comorbidity between SUDs and other psychiatric disorders. At least four hypotheses have been proposed to explain this overlap: 1) a common set of genes increases risk for multiple disorders; 2) a common set of environmental factors increases risk for multiple disorders; 3) psychiatric disorders increase risk for substance abuse through a phenotypic basis (e.g., individuals who are anxious or depressed use substances for symptom relief); and 4) other disorders develop as a consequence of substance abuse (e.g., anxiety and depressive disorders due to changes in the brain associated with long term drug exposure).

Several large-scale family and twin studies have addressed the basis for this comorbidity. The results have varied somewhat, but evidence is accumulating that genetic factors increase risk to both addictive and psychiatric disorders, and that different genetic factors are disorder-specific (e.g., Kendler et al. 2003b). Environmental factors are also important, but there is little evidence that family environmental factors are involved.

These results are consistent with findings from genetic association studies. As is noted in other chapters in this volume, the candidate genes associated with SUDs are also implicated in many other psychiatric disorders. Some association studies of SUDs have found risk alleles only in subgroups defined by comorbid psychiatric disorders, such as the association between 5HTTLPR and antisocial alcoholism described previously. There is also evidence from linkage studies that specific loci contribute to both psychiatric and substance use disorders. A recent report suggests that some of the genetic overlap for alcoholism and major depression in the COGA study described previously is due to variation in the M_2 muscarinic acetylcholine receptor (Wang et al. 2004).

As the results continue to accumulate from molecular genetic studies, our understanding of the mechanisms underlying comorbidity should become clearer. It is also important to recognize that there are likely to be multiple mechanisms involved in these processes because there are multiple pathways to addiction. For some individuals, genetic risk may contribute to comorbidity because of genetic influences on a primary SUD, from which psychiatric illness develops. For others genetic risk for an SUD may be indirect, arising through a primary psychiatric disorder.

Conclusion

Evidence regarding genetic influences on substance use disorders has accumulated rapidly in the past decade. Despite the obvious volitional component of substance use, genetic effects on SUDs are as strong as for any other common psychiatric disorder. It appears that these genetic effects are not completely substance-specific but that there is substantial overlap of genetic influence across different substances and also across SUDs and other psychiatric disorders. Identification of specific genes will advance our understanding of the mechanisms by which genetic vulnerability develops into an SUD and the basis for SUD comorbidity.

The results from genetic studies of SUDs reinforce the observation that family members of an affected individual are at increased risk for developing problems with that substance and with substances from other classes. Individuals with a strong family history should be counseled about their risk and the need to be cautious about their substance use.

Identification of specific genes is just the first step. The next step will entail the difficult task of understanding how susceptibility loci combine with each other and with experiences during the course of development to produce SUDs. As suggested by animal studies, it is likely that there will be partially independent genetic influences on component processes, such as sensitivity, craving, tolerance, and withdrawal. This level of knowledge will enable the development of more effective pharmacological interventions that can be targeted to individuals based on their genotypes. In recent years the technologies for identifying genes and measuring gene action have advanced rapidly. The task for genetic researchers in the years to come is to incorporate measured genes into comprehensive theories for the development of SUDs.

References

Ball D, Collier D: Substance misuse, in Psychiatric Genetics and Genomics. Edited by McGuffin P, Owen MJ, Gottesman II. Oxford, England, Oxford University Press, 2002, pp 267–302

Batra V, Patkar AA, Berrettini WH, et al: The genetic determinants of smoking. Chest 123:1730–1739, 2003

Bierut LJ, Rice JP, Goate A, et al: A genomic scan for habitual smoking in families of alcoholics: common and specific genetic factors in substance dependence. Am J Med Genet 124A:19–27, 2004

Blum K, Noble EP, Sheridan P, et al: Association of the A1 allele of the D2 dopamine receptor gene with severe alcoholism. Alcohol 8:409–416, 1991

Bohman M, Sigvardsson S, Cloninger CR: Maternal inheritance of alcohol abuse: cross-fostering analysis of adopted women. Arch Gen Psychiatry 38:965–969, 1981

Cadoret RJ, O'Gorman TW, Troughton E, et al: Alcoholism and antisocial personality: interrelationships, genetic and environmental factors. Arch Gen Psychiatry 42:161–167, 1985

Cadoret RJ, Troughton E, O'Gorman TW: Genetic and environmental factors in alcohol abuse and antisocial personality. J Stud Alcohol 48:1–8, 1987

Cloninger CR, Bohman M, Sigvardsson S: Inheritance of alcohol abuse: cross-fostering analysis of adopted men. Arch Gen Psychiatry 38:861–868, 1981

Cotton NS: The familial incidence of alcoholism: a review. J Stud Alcohol 40:89–116, 1979

Crabbe JC: Alcohol and genetics: new models. Am J Med Genet 114:969–974, 2002

Dick DM, Foroud T: Candidate genes for alcohol dependence: a review of genetic evidence from human studies. Alcohol Clin Exp Res 27:868–879, 2003

Ehlers CL, Gilder DA, Wall TL, et al: Genomic screen for loci associated with alcohol dependence in Mission Indians. Am J Med Genet Neuropsychiatr Genet 128B:110–115, 2004

Foroud T, Edenberg HJ, Goate A, et al: Alcoholism susceptibility loci: confirmation studies in a replicate sample and further mapping. Alcohol Clin Exp Res 24:933–945, 2000

Goodwin DW, Schulsinger F, Hermansen L, et al: Alcohol problems in adoptees raised apart from alcoholic parents. Arch Gen Psychiatry 28:238–243, 1973

Goodwin DW, Schulsinger F, Knop J, et al: Psychopathology in adopted and nonadopted daughters of alcoholics. Arch Gen Psychiatry 34:1005–1009, 1977

Gynther LM, Carey G, Gottesman II, et al: A twin study of non-alcohol substance abuse. Psychiatry Res 56:213–220, 1995

Heath AC, Bucholz KK, Madden PAF, et al: Genetic and environmental contributions to alcohol dependence risk in a national twin sample: consistency of findings in women and men. Psychol Med 27:1381–1396, 1997

Heath AC, Madden PA, Martin NG: Statistical methods in genetic research on smoking. Stat Methods Med Res 7:165–186, 1998

Hill SY, Shen S, Zezza N, et al: A genome wide search for alcoholism susceptibility genes. Am J Med Genet Neuropsychiatr Genet 128B:102–113, 2004

Kaij L: Alcoholism in Twins. Stockholm, Almqvist & Wiksell, 1960

Kendler KS, Karkowski LM, Corey LA, et al: Genetic and environmental risk factors in the aetiology of drug initiation and subsequent misuse in women. Br J Psychiatry 175:351–356, 1999a

Kendler KS, Neale MC, Sullivan PF, et al: A population-based twin study in women of smoking initiation and nicotine dependence. Psychol Med 29:299–308, 1999b

Kendler KS, Karkowski LM, Pedersen NL: Tobacco consumption in Swedish twins reared apart and reared together. Arch Gen Psychiatry 57:886–892, 2000

Kendler KS, Jacobson KJ, Prescott CA: Specificity of genetic and environmental risk factors for use and abuse of cannabis, cocaine, hallucinogens, sedatives, stimulants, and opiates in male twins. Am J Psychiatry 160:687–695, 2003a

Kendler KS, Prescott CA, Myers J, et al: The structure of genetic and environmental risk factors for common psychiatric and substance use disorders in men and women. Arch Gen Psychiatry 60:929–937, 2003b

Kessler RC, Crum RM, Warner LA, et al: Lifetime co-occurrence of DSM-III-R alcohol abuse and dependence with other psychiatric disorders in the National Comorbidity Survey. Arch Gen Psychiatry 54:313–320, 1997

Kreek MJ, Nilesen DZ, LaForge KS: Genes associated with addiction: alcoholism, opiate and cocaine addiction. Neuromolecular Med 5:85–108, 2004

Langbehn DR, Cadoret RJ, Caspers K, et al: Genetic and environmental risk factors for the onset of drug use and problems in adoptees. Drug Alcohol Depend 69:151–167, 2003

Lerman C, Berrettini W: Elucidating the role of genetic factors in smoking behavior and nicotine dependence. Am J Med Genet 118B:48–54, 2003

Li MD: The genetics of smoking related behavior: a brief review. Am J Med Sci 326:168–173, 2003

Long JC, Knowler WC, Hanson RL, et al: Evidence for genetic linkage to alcohol dependence on chromosomes 4 and 11 from an autosome-wide scan in an American Indian population. Am J Med Genet 81:216–221, 1998

Madden PA, Pedersen NL, Kaprio J, et al: The epidemiology and genetics of smoking initiation and persistence: cross-cultural comparisons of twin study results. Twin Res 7:82–97, 2004

Maes HH, Sullivan PF, Bulik CM, et al: A twin study of genetic and environmental influences on tobacco initiation, regular tobacco use and nicotine dependence. Psychol Med 34:1251–1261, 2004

McGue M, Pickens RW, Svikis DS: Sex and age effects on the inheritance of alcohol problems: a twin study. J Abnorm Psychol 101:3–17, 1992

Merikangas KR, Stolar M, Stevens DE: Familial transmission of substance use disorders. Arch Gen Psychiatry 55:973–979, 1998

Nurnberger JI, Foroud T, Flury L, et al: Evidence for a locus on chromosome 1 that influences vulnerability to alcoholism and affective disorder. Am J Psychiatry 158:718–724, 2001

Prescott CA: The genetic epidemiology of alcoholism: sex differences and future directions, in Alcohol in Health and Disease. Edited by Agarwal DP, Seitz HK. New York, Marcel Dekker, 2001, pp 125–149

Prescott CA, Aggen SH, Kendler KS: Sex differences in the sources of genetic liability to alcohol abuse and dependence in a population based sample of U.S. twins. Alcohol Clin Exp Res 23:1136–1144, 1999

Prescott CA, Caldwell CB, Carey G, et al: The Washington University Twin Study of Alcoholism. Am J Med Genet Neuropsychiatr Genet 2005

Prescott CA, Sullivan PF, Webb T, et al: Linkage of alcohol dependence symptoms to chromosome 4 in the Irish Affected Sib Pair Study of Alcohol Dependence. Am J Med Genet Neuropsychiatr Genet (in press)

Rice DP: Economic costs of substance abuse, 1995. Proc Assoc Am Physicians 111:119–125, 1999

Roe A, Burks B: Adult adjustment of foster children of alcoholic and psychotic parentage and the influence of the foster home. Memoirs of the Section on Alcohol Studies, No 3. New Haven, CT, Yale University, 1945

Room R, Graham K, Rehn J, et al: Drinking and its burden in a global perspective: policy considerations and options. Eur Addiction Res 9: 165–175, 2003

Saccone NL, Goode EL, Bergen AW: Genetic Analysis Workshop 13: summary of analyses of alcohol and cigarette use phenotypes in the Framingham Heart Study. Genet Epidemiol 25(suppl):S90–S97, 2003

Sigvardsson S, Bohman M, Cloninger CR: Replication of the Stockholm Adoption Study of Alcoholism: confirmatory cross-fostering analysis. Arch Gen Psychiatry 53:681–687, 1996

Straub RE, Sullivan PF, Ma Y, et al: Susceptibility genes for nicotine dependence: a genome scan and followup in an independent sample suggest that regions on chromosomes 2, 4, 10, 16, 17 and 18 merit further study. Mol Psychiatry 4:129–144, 1999

Sullivan PF, Kendler KS: The genetic epidemiology of smoking. Nicotine Tobacco Res 1(suppl):S51-S57, 1997

True WR, Heath AC, Bucholz K, et al: Models of treatment seeking for alcoholism: the role of genes and environment. Alcohol Clin Exp Res 20:1577–1581, 1996

Tsuang MT, Lyons M, Eisen SA, et al: Genetic influences on DSM-III-R drug abuse and dependence: a study of 3,372 twin pairs. Am J Med Genet 67:473–477, 1996

Tsuang MT, Lyons MK, Meyer JM, et al: Co-occurrence of abuse of different drugs in men: the role of drug-specific and shared vulnerabilities. Arch Gen Psychiatry 55:967–972, 1998

Uhl GR, Liu QR, Naiman D: Substance abuse vulnerability loci: converging genome scanning data. Trends Genet 18:420–425, 2002

van den Bree MB, Svikis DS, Pickens RW: Genetic influences in antisocial personality and drug use disorders. Drug Alcohol Depend 49:177–187, 1998

Vink JM, Beem AL, Posthuma D, et al: Linkage analysis of smoking initiation and quantity in Dutch sibling pairs. Pharmacogenomics J 4:274–282, 2004

Wang JC, Hinrichs AL, Stock H, et al: Evidence of common and specific genetic effects: association of the muscarinic acetylcholine receptor M2 (CHRM2) gene with alcohol dependence and major depressive syndrome. Hum Mol Genet 13:1903–1911, 2004

Chapter 6

Genetic Influence on the Development of Antisocial Behavior

Kristen C. Jacobson, Ph.D.

Antisocial behavior is studied by virtually every field of social science, including psychology, sociology, epidemiology, and criminology, as well as psychiatry. Discussions concerning the complex interplay between genes and environments are therefore of interest to researchers across many domains. Although each field has its own particular ways of assessing antisocial behavior, there is a strong correlation between different measures. For example, in recent versions of the American Psychiatric Association's *Diagnostic and Statistical Manual of Mental Disorders* (DSM) (American Psychiatric Association 1987, 1994, 2000), a diagnosis of adult antisocial personality disorder (ASPD) is given only if the individual also meets criteria for earlier child and adolescent conduct disorder. Psychiatrists and psychologists have recognized that criminal behavior may be preceded by other psychiatric disorders, such as attention-deficit disorder and conduct disorder in childhood (Mannuzza et al. 1989; Satterfield et al. 1982). The majority of adult criminals are also thought to have ASPD, although this is partly due to the fact that committing illegal activities is one of the diagnostic criteria for ASPD.

Many measures of adolescent delinquent and aggressive behavior contain items similar to those found in DSM-III-R and DSM-IV criteria for conduct disorder. Because of the strong correlation across different measures of antisocial behavior, I focus here on genetic and environmental influences on antisocial behavior, broadly defined. One notable exception is that I omit discussion of attention-deficit/hyperactivity disorder (ADHD). Although there is evidence that ADHD may be related to conduct disorder, the fact that there may be specific genetic influence governing the more cognitive processes of inattention (e.g., Faraone et al. 2000; Silberg et al. 1996b) means that extrapolation from results of behavioral genetic studies of ADHD may be misleading.

In contrast to findings from studies of many other phenotypes, when taken as a whole, results from behavioral genetic research on antisocial behavior are often inconsistent across studies. Although there is strong evidence of at least some degree of genetic influence on individual differences in antisocial behavior, overall estimates of heritability (i.e., the proportion of variation due to genetic factors) can vary substantially across studies, from zero influence to .90, and appear to be influenced by a multitude of methodological and substantive factors, including sample age, the rater (e.g., self-report versus maternal ratings), and developmental heterogeneity. Also in question is the extent to which between-family environmental factors (i.e., shared environments) impact on individual differences in antisocial behavior.

In this chapter, I attempt to bring some sort of rhyme and reason to the underlying inconsistencies across studies. The chapter begins with a simple overview and comparison of results from twin and adoption studies of antisocial behavior divided into three different developmental epochs (early childhood, adolescence, and adulthood). I then discuss results from the handful of longitudinal and quasi-longitudinal behavioral genetic studies regarding genetic influences on stability and change in antisocial behavior. It should be noted that time and space constraints limit the number of studies that can be reviewed, so the focus of this chapter is primarily on general trends derived from population-based samples. However, in a recent review article of the genetics of antisocial behavior, Slutske (2001) reported that there are more than 100 published twin and adoption studies of antisocial behavior. Interested readers are encouraged to consult this brief review, as well as to read results from different meta-analyses of antisocial behavior that try to account for some of the systematic variation in results across studies (e.g., Miles and Carey 1997; Rhee and Waldman 2002).

In the second part of the chapter, I discuss factors that may account for heterogeneity of results across studies. These factors include methodological artifacts, such as different raters, as well as potentially theoretical reasons for actually expecting observed heterogeneity of genetic influence, such as the effects of age on expression of genetic and environmental influence, and evidence for different developmental trajectories of antisocial behavior across the life span.

Finally, I conclude the chapter by discussing one of the most exciting new areas of research—the role of gene × environment interactions in the development of antisocial behavior—which promises to make our understanding of genetic and environmental influences on antisocial behavior even more complex.

Genetic Influence on Developmental Epochs

Problem Behavior in Early Childhood

There is reasonably compelling and consistent evidence for genetic influences on early childhood aggression and problem behaviors, although the absolute magnitude of this influence varies across studies (and sometimes within a study). For example, in one of the earlier studies of problem behavior in young childhood, Ghodsian-Carpey and Baker (1987) reported wide-ranging heritabilities of .24 to .94 for maternal ratings of different indicators of aggressive behavior among 4- to 7-year-old twins. With the exception of a small study of 229 Colorado preschool twin pairs (Schmitz et al. 1994), which found only limited evidence for genetic influence on antisocial behavior, the majority of other studies using maternal ratings of early childhood problem behavior have reported heritability estimates in the range of .50 to .60 (e.g., Bartels et al. 2004; van den Oord and Rowe 1997; van den Oord et al. 1996). In one of the few studies using child self-report, Arsenault et al. (2003) used an innovative interview, the Berkeley Puppet Interview, to obtain self-reports from 5-year-old children on their own hostile/aggressive, conduct-disordered, and oppositional behavior. In a univariate analysis of a composite measure of these three behaviors, heritability was estimated at .30, with a nonsignificant shared environmental influence of .10. Thus, results from behavioral genetic studies of problem behavior in early childhood are, with only one major exception (i.e., the Schmitz et al. 1994 study), largely in agreement that genetic factors are important for individual differences in problem behavior, with most studies showing estimates of moderately high heritabilities (.50–.60).

Late Childhood and Adolescent Antisocial Behavior

Delinquency and Conduct Disorder

In contrast to studies of problem behavior in early childhood, there is considerable evidence that genetic influences are weaker, and shared environmental influences are stronger, for late childhood and adolescent delinquent or conduct-disordered behavior. In one of the first twin studies of adolescent self-reports of antisocial behavior (including items assessing minor delinquency, theft, and aggression) from approximately 265 same-sex American twin pairs, Rowe (1983) concluded that both genetic and shared environmental factors may contribute to adolescent delinquency.

More recent studies using large-scale population-based samples have also concluded that genes and environments each account for between 20% and 25% of the variation in adolescent self-reported delinquency and conduct problems (e.g., Eaves et al. 1997; Taylor et al. 2000). In addition, at least three published twin studies have examined genetic and environmental influences on adult retrospective reports of conduct disorder. Two of the studies found nearly identical results among males. In the earlier study of male twins from the Vietnam Era Twin Registry, Lyons et al. (1995) reported only a modest heritability of .07, and a shared environmental influence of .31, for conduct-disordered behavior prior to age 15. Among male twins from the Virginia Twin Registry, Jacobson et al. (2002), reported estimates of .06 and .28, respectively, for genetic and shared environmental influences on conduct-disordered behavior prior to age 15, although heritability was higher, and shared environmental influences were lower, among females. The third study (Slutske et al. 1997), using adult twin data from the Australian Twin Register, may be viewed as an outlier, as the heritability for conduct disorder under the best-fitting model was much higher than in other studies (.71) for both males and females, and shared environmental influences were zero.

Studies of maternal ratings of adolescent delinquency and conduct-disordered behavior also report strong evidence for both significant genetic and shared environmental influences, with estimates for genetic factors typically ranging from .20 to .50, and estimates of shared environmental influences ranging from .30 to .40 (Edelbrock et al. 1995; Eley et al. 1999; Thapar and McGuffin 1996).

Finally, a handful of adoption and twin-sibling studies have examined genetic and environmental influences on problem behavior in adolescence. Results from these studies are somewhat less consistent. For one of the studies, based on a sample of adolescents in the Iowa Adoption Study, results suggested a complete absence of genetic influence on variation in antisocial behavior (Cadoret 1978). Specifically, this study found virtually identical rates of psychiatric disorders among children with antisocial biological background (25%) and control subjects (27%); this finding indicates that the presence of a biological (genetic) risk for antisocial behavior was not related to greater likelihood of antisocial behavior compared with a lack of a family history of antisocial behavior. In contrast, in the second study, based on a sample of 172 adoptive and biological twin pairs from the Colorado Adoption Project, Deater-Deckard and Plomin (1999) reported significant influences on both genetic (.36) and shared environmental (.22) influences on maternal ratings of delinquent behavior. Different still are results from the third study, based on data from twin, full siblings, half-siblings, and unrelated siblings in the Nonshared Environment and Adolescent Development Project, which reported fairly high estimates of heritability (.63–.66) and little evidence for shared environmental factors (Neiderhiser et al. 1996). In conclusion, although many studies of adolescent delinquency find stronger shared environmental influences and weaker genetic influences than studies of problem behaviors in young children, there is inconsistency across studies.

Aggressive Behavior

One of the factors that might account for differences in estimates of heritability and shared environmental influences on antisocial behavior in late childhood and adolescence is whether studies focused on aggressive antisocial behavior, nonaggressive antisocial behavior, or a measure combining both aggressive and nonaggressive behaviors. Specifically, there is accumulating evidence that aggressive behavior in late childhood and adolescence has a stronger genetic component than nonaggressive delinquent or conduct-disordered behavior. For example, at least three published studies using parental reports on the Child Behavior Checklist (CBCL; Achenbach and Edelbrock 1979) examined differences in heritability for the Aggressive versus Delinquent Behavior subscales. All three of these studies reported substantially higher estimates of heritability (range = .60–.80) for aggressive behaviors than for nonaggressive delinquent behaviors (range = .30–.60; Edelbrock et al. 1995; Eley et al. 1999; Gjone and Stevenson 1997). In addition, two of these studies reported that shared environmental factors did not significantly influence twin similarity for aggressive behavior, although they explained between 27% and 64% of the variation in delinquent behavior (see Edelbrock et al. 1995; Eley et al. 1999). What is remarkable about these results is the overall similarity of pattern across studies, especially since the results were based on data from eight different birth cohorts across four different countries (Sweden, Britain, Norway, and United States).

To test the hypothesis that more severe aggressive or psychopathological behavior is more heritable than nonaggressive antisocial behavior, we recently fitted multivariate behavioral genetic models to antisocial data from 9- to 10-year-old twins in the University of Southern California (USC) Risk Factors for Antisocial Behavior Study (K. C. Jacobson, L. Baker, A. Raine, manuscript in preparation, 2005). Figure 6–1 presents this model, which was fitted to maternal ratings on five different indices of antisocial behavior: 1) Aggressive (AGG) and 2) Delinquent (DEL) subscales of the CBCL (Achenbach and Edelbrock 1979); 3) ratings of conduct disorder symptoms from the Diagnostic Interview Schedule for Children (DISC; Costello et al. 1985); 4) a newly developed

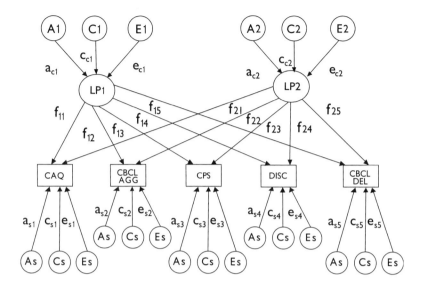

Figure 6–1. Multivariate behavioral genetic model for covariation across five measures of antisocial behavior.

CAQ=Child Aggression Questionnaire; CBCL=Child Behavior Checklist (AGG=Aggression subscale; DEL=Delinquent Behavior subscale); CPS=Child Psychopathy Scale; DISC=Diagnostic Interview Schedule for Children. A=additive genetic influence; C=shared environmental influence; E = non-shared environmental influence; LP1=first latent factor; LP2=second latent factor. Subscript c represents genetic and environmental influences that are common across the five measures and operate through the latent phenotypes. In contrast, subscript s denotes genetic and environmental influences that are specific to each variable. Parameters f11–f15 through f21–f25 represent the factor loadings for each of the two latent factors.

questionnaire, the Childhood Aggression Questionnaire (CAQ; A. Raine, K. Dodge, R. Loeber, et al., manuscript under review, 2005); and 5) the Child Psychopathy Scale (CPS; Lynam 1997). These measured variables are represented by the rectangles in Figure 6–1.

The model shown assumes that there are two underlying latent phenotypes (i.e., factors)—latent factors LP1 and LP2—that account for the correlations across the five different measures. Arrows from the latent phenotypes to the measured variables represent factor loadings (f_{11}–f_{15} for Factor 1; f_{21}–f_{25} for Factor 2).

Variation in these latent phenotypes, in turn, is accounted for by a common set of genetic and of shared and nonshared environmental influences (A1, C1, and E1, respectively, for Factor 1, and A2, C2, and E2, respectively, for Factor 2). The proportion of variation in each of the factors due to these genetic and environmental influences is obtained by squaring each of the respective parameter estimates (i.e., a_{c1}, c_{c1}, e_{c1}, and a_{c2}, c_{c2}, e_{c2}). In addition to modeling variation in the measured variables that is due to the underlying latent phenotypes, this approach also allows for specific genetic, shared, and nonshared environmental influences on each of the measured variables that are not shared with genetic and environmental influences on the other variables (i.e., a_{s1}–e_{s5}). The two-factor model shown in Figure 6–1 was tested against an alternative model in which all of the covariation across measures could be accounted for by a single underlying latent phenotype. This latter model tested the hypothesis that all five measures of antisocial behavior represented a single, unitary construct.

Preliminary analyses of both the same-sex male and same-sex female twins strongly indicated the presence of two distinct, underlying latent factors that account for the correlation across measures. Figure 6–2 presents the results from the analysis of the female twins. For simplicity, the specific genetic and environmental influences are not shown, as they relate to genetic and environmental variation in each of the five measures that is not shared with the other measures. Dashed lines represent parameter estimates that are not significantly different from zero. As can be seen in this figure, the first factor (LP1) was defined by significant factor loadings (range=.50 to .99) on all five measures of antisocial behavior. This suggests the presence of a "general deviance" factor, which accounts for 25% to over 90% of the variance in each measure. In contrast, the second factor (LP2) loaded significantly on only the two measures of aggression and the CPS, indicating that it may be tapping more severe aggressive and psychopathic behavior that is not shared with a general deviance factor. This factor accounted for 20%–36% of the variance in these three measures.

Figure 6–2 also shows the genetic and environmental contributions to variation in these underlying latent phenotypes. As can be

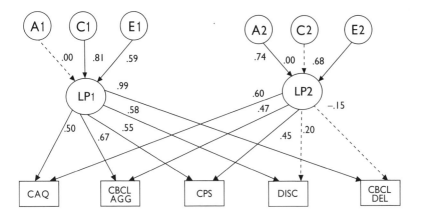

Figure 6–2. Standardized parameter estimates for genetic and environmental factor loadings on five measures of antisocial behavior for female-female twins.

CAQ=Child Aggression Questionnaire; CBCL=Child Behavior Checklist (AGG=Aggression subscale; DEL=Delinquent Behavior subscale); CPS=Child Psychopathy Scale; DISC=Diagnostic Interview Schedule for Children. A=additive genetic influence; C=shared environmental influence; E = nonshared environmental influence; LP1=first latent factor; LP2=second latent factor. Dashed lines represent parameter estimates that are not significantly different from zero.

seen very clearly in these results for female-female twins, the pattern of genetic and environmental influence on variation differed dramatically across the two different underlying latent phenotypes. Specifically, for Factor 1, the general deviance factor, all of the variation could be accounted for by environmental factors. Shared environmental factors accounted for approximately 65% of the variance (.81×.81), and nonshared environmental factors accounted for the remaining 35% (.59×.59). In contrast, the heritability of the aggressive-psychopathology factor (LP2) was estimated at approximately 54% (.74×.74), and nonshared environmental influences accounted for the remaining 46% of the variance in this factor (.68 ×.68).

Moreover, although the phenotypic structure of the first general deviance factor was similar for males and females, the absolute magnitude of genetic and environmental influences on this underlying factor varied across sex. In particular, among males, genetic factors accounted for 49% of the variance in this underlying factor (results not shown), although the heritability was estimated to be zero among females. Conversely, shared environmental influences on variation in this underlying latent factor were stronger for females (64%) than for males (40%). In contrast, not only was the phenotypic factor structure of the second, aggressive-psychopathology factor similar across males and females, but genetic and environmental influences on this second latent factor were virtually identical across sexes, with genetic and nonshared environmental factors each accounting for approximately one-half the variation. Results from these preliminary analyses support the hypothesis that general problem behavior is more strongly influenced by environmental factors, whereas aggressive, pathological antisocial behavior is more strongly influenced by genetic factors.

Adult Antisocial Behavior and Criminality

In contrast to the somewhat inconsistent results for genetic influence on adolescent antisocial behavior, results from twin and adoption studies of adults are nearly unanimous in support of the hypothesis that aggressive and criminal behavior have a fairly substantial genetic component (see Brennan and Mednick 1993 and DiLalla and Gottesman 1989 for reviews of the earlier literature, and Rhee and Waldman 2002 for a more recent review and meta-analysis). For example, on the basis of data from the Danish Adoption Registry, it was found that the average rate of criminal convictions among male adoptees with neither biological nor adoptive parent convictions was 13.5%. When adoptive parents, but not biological parents, had criminal convictions, the rate of criminality among adoptees increased to only 14.7%. In contrast, the rate of criminal convictions when biological parents, but not adoptive parents, had criminal convictions increased to 20.0% (Brennan and Mednick 1993; Mednick et al. 1984).

Thus, biological (genetic) risk, but not environmental risk, was associated with a higher incidence of criminal convictions, supporting the notion of genetic influence on adult antisocial behavior. Similar findings for high heritability of adult antisocial behavior have been reported in other adoption (e.g., Cadoret 1978) and twin (e.g., Cloninger and Gottesman 1997; Jacobson et al. 2002; Lyons et al. 1995) samples. Thus, for behavioral genetic investigations of adult antisocial behavior, most studies find evidence for heritabilities between .40 and .60. Moreover, the results from twin studies suggest that the importance of shared environmental influences on individual differences in adult antisocial behavior is negligible.

Differences in Heritability of Antisocial Behavior Over Time

Thus far, I have presented results from a variety of twin and adoption studies of antisocial behavior at different developmental periods. Although there is considerable variation across studies in terms of the actual magnitude of genetic and environmental factors, at least two general patterns emerge: 1) genetic influence increases from adolescence to adulthood, and 2) environmental influences appear to be the most important factor in accounting for variation in antisocial behavior during the adolescent years. However, drawing conclusions about developmental changes in the relative influence of genetic and shared environmental factors on antisocial behavior from cross-study comparisons is problematic, because studies use different samples and different measures of antisocial behavior. These differences in methodologies may introduce systematic biases.

To circumvent these possible biases, at least two meta-analyses have been conducted to statistically test for differences in genetic and environmental influences across age while controlling for potential differences across study in sample and methodology. In the first study, which focused on studies of aggressive antisocial behaviors, Miles and Carey (1997) concluded that although juvenile aggressive behavior was influenced equally by both genetic and shared environmental factors (each accounting for approximately 20% of the variance), genetic influences on adult aggressive behavior were markedly higher (40%) and shared environmental influences were negligible. The second study, which reviewed 51 twin and adoption studies of both aggressive and nonaggressive behavior, also found evidence of significant age differences (Rhee and Waldman 2002). However, in these authors' analysis, the primary difference was in the effect of the shared environment. Among studies of children and adolescents, shared environmental effects accounted for 16%–20% of the variance, compared with estimates of only 9% among studies of adults. Genetic factors, in contrast, accounted for 41%–46% of the variance at all ages.

Although meta-analyses can account for some of the factors that may bias cross-sectional comparisons, the best way of estimating changes in the relative importance of genetic and environmental influences on antisocial behavior over time is to rely on data that assesses antisocial behavior from the same sample of twins at two or more different ages. At least two, large-scale, quasi-longitudinal twin studies have examined the question of age-related changes in heritability estimates, and both studies reported remarkably consistent evidence for significant changes in the heritability of antisocial behavior across age. In the first study, using retrospective data from adult male-male twins in the Vietnam Twin Registry, Lyons et al. (1995) found that heritability increased from .07 for antisocial behavior assessed prior to age 15 (juvenile antisocial behavior) to .43 for antisocial behavior assessed at ages 15 and older (adult antisocial behavior). Conversely, shared environmental influences explained 31% of the variation in juvenile antisocial traits but only 5% of the variation in adult antisocial traits (Lyons et al. 1995). The second study, based on an analysis of retrospective reports of child, adolescent, and adult antisocial behavior that drew on data from both male and female twin pairs from the Virginia Twin Registry, also found evidence for increasing genetic effects and decreasing shared environmental effects, especially among males (Jacobson et al. 2002). Among males, heritability increased from .06 to .40, and shared environmental influences decreased from .28 to .11. Among females, the difference in heritability was less marked (.29 to .42), but still showed a pattern of increasing genetic effects across age.

Thus, taken together, studies suggest that there is systematic heterogeneity across age in estimates of the overall magnitude of genetic and shared environmental factors. These findings are consistent with the patterns of increasing heritability and decreasing effects of shared environment with age that have been observed in studies of other phenotypes, such as personality and cognition (see Plomin 1986 for review). These patterns suggest that effects of shared family, community, and neighborhood characteristics that influence antisocial behavior during adolescence may have little continuing influence on adult antisocial behavior.

Genetic and Environmental Influences on Continuity and Change in Antisocial Behavior

Longitudinal Behavioral Genetic Studies

In addition to estimating more reliably the potential changes in the magnitude of genetic and environmental influences on antisocial behavior over time, longitudinal behavioral genetic studies can tell us the extent to which genetic and environmental factors contribute to *continuity and change* in antisocial behavior over time. When different manifestations of antisocial behavior across developmental periods are considered, psychiatrists, psychologists, and criminologists are mainly in agreement that there is remarkable phenotypic stability to antisocial behavior.

In a seminal study using data from four longitudinal studies of males, Robins (1978) concluded that although most children with antisocial behavior problems do not become antisocial adults, virtually all adults with antisocial behavior problems were antisocial children. What is particularly remarkable about this result is that it was replicated in four independent samples, even though the samples represented males from different racial and social backgrounds and from different historical eras (Robins 1978). Childhood behaviors were more predictive of adult antisocial behavior than family variables, including parental antisocial behavior, family structure, and social class.

Following this landmark report, there have been dozens of studies demonstrating a strong continuity between child, adolescent, and adult antisocial behaviors. For example, rates of adult criminal convictions are higher among samples of individuals diagnosed with ADHD compared with control groups (Mannuzza et al. 1989; Satterfield et al. 1982), and attention problems, impulsivity, and activity have been found to be precursors to later antisocial behavior (Loeber and Hay 1991). Likewise, aggressive behavior in childhood has also been found to predict delinquent and criminal behavior during adolescence and young adulthood. For instance, in a follow-up study of more than 1,000 subjects from a cohort of 10-year-olds in Sweden, Stattin and Magnusson (1989) reported that teacher ratings of aggression at age 13 predicted conviction by age 26, particularly multiple convictions. Finally, childhood ADHD and conduct disorder predict adult ASPD and criminality (e.g., Simonoff et al. 2004).

Developmental Behavioral Genetic Studies

Although the studies summarized above provide evidence for a strong phenotypic continuity of antisocial behavior, they cannot tell us *why* there is stability of behavior over time. Understanding the mechanisms behind both stability and change in antisocial behavior is of particular importance to clinicians, since any plans for prevention need to incorporate the processes through which antisocial children turn into antisocial adolescent and adults. Developmental behavioral genetic studies are a means of investigating the *sources* of developmental stability and change in behavior—that is, the extent to which genes and environments contribute to continuity and change. In this type of study, genetically informative kin are interviewed or observed on more than one occasion, and genetic influence on continuity and change is estimated from the pattern of cross-twin, cross-time correlations. Although longitudinal samples of this type are rare, inspection of the results from the existing published studies reveals some interesting patterns.

Sources of Stability in Antisocial Behavior Across Childhood and Adolescence

In one of the first developmental behavioral genetic studies of antisocial behavior, van den Oord and Rowe (1997) examined the developmental stability of problem behavior, including antisocial behavior, in a study of full siblings, half siblings, and cousins from ages 4–6 to 6–8 to 8–10 years. The authors concluded that there was substantial evidence of a genetic effect on the stability of problem behavior, because the cross-time sibling correlation was higher among full sibling pairs (who share, on average, 50% of their segregating genes) than among half siblings (who share only 25% of their segregating genes). Structural equation models revealed a moderate correlation of antisocial behavior across waves ($r = .57$). Of this stability, 46% of the correlation could be attributable to genetic influences, and the remaining 54% was attributed to shared environmental influences.

Other evidence for genetic influence on the continuity of antisocial behavior across childhood and early adolescence comes from a large body of research using longitudinal data from a sample drawn from The Netherlands Twin Registry. In this study, assessments of problem behavior using the maternal reports of the CBCL were obtained at ages 3, 7, 10, and 12. In one of the most recent and comprehensive analyses from this sample, Bartels et al. (2004) reported across-time correlations for maternal reports of CBCL Externalizing symptoms ranging from .46 to .76, demonstrating remarkable stability of antisocial behavior across age. Moreover, these phenotypic correlations from age 3 to age 12 were explained predominantly by both genetic and shared environmental factors.

Evidence for a genetic basis for stability of antisocial behavior across adolescence has also been found (Eley et al. 2003; O'Connor et al. 1998). In the first longitudinal study of 405 twin and sibling pairs from the Nonshared Environment and Adolescent Development Project, O'Connor et al. (1998) found that genetic factors accounted for over 50% of the phenotypic continuity of antisocial behavior symptoms from ages 10 to 18. Interestingly, one of the few studies to examine genetic and environmental influences on aggressive versus nonaggressive delinquent behavior found evidence for a slightly different pattern of genetic and environmental influences on continuity of antisocial behavior from childhood (ages 8–9) to adolescence (ages 13–14) (Eley et al. 2003). Specifically, continuity in aggressive behavior was attributed almost entirely to genetic factors (accounting for 84% of the phenotypic correlation). In contrast, both genetic (44%) and shared environmental (54%) influences accounted for the stability in nonaggressive delinquent behaviors.

Sources of Stability in Antisocial Behavior From Adolescence to Adulthood

As of this writing, there are no published studies of change in antisocial behavior between childhood and adulthood using prospective, genetically informative samples. This is unfortunate, given the dramatic differences in heritability estimates that appear in a comparison of cross-sectional research. Nevertheless, two published studies using population-based twin samples have been able to examine the genetic and environmental influences on stability and change across antisocial behavior from childhood to adolescence by using retrospective reports of juvenile antisocial behavior and retrospective/current reports of adult antisocial behavior. In both studies, genetic factors accounted for 20%–50% of the correlations among juvenile and adult antisocial behaviors, and shared environmental factors accounted for 6%–40% of these correlations. It is especially interesting that even though shared environmental factors had only a negligible influence on adult antisocial behavior in these studies (less than 10% of the variance), these same factors appeared to explain the continuity of antisocial behavior from adolescence to adulthood.

Factors Accounting for Change in Antisocial Behavior

Results from the foregoing longitudinal studies point to significant genetic effects on continuity in problem behavior, both within and across developmental epoch. Shared environmental factors are also implicated, especially with respect to continuities of childhood antisocial behavior. In addition, some, but not all, of these studies provide evidence for the appearance of age-specific genetic effects on antisocial behavior, indicating that genetic factors may also account for *change* in antisocial behavior. Although an individual's DNA is present at birth and does not change throughout the life span, it is possible for studies to reveal the presence of "new" genetic effects on behavior. The appearance of the new genetic effects can stem from a variety of sources, including significant biological changes (e.g., puberty) that may "turn on or off" genes or from changes in the social environment that may either enhance or suppress genetic influences on behavior.

Interestingly, in contrast to the remarkable consistency in results for *stability* of genetic influence over time, studies vary greatly in their evidence for *new* genetic effects. For example, in the van den Oord and Rowe (1997) study, the influence of new genetic factors did not appear at any point in their assessments from ages 4–6 to 8–10. In contrast, Bartels et al. (2004) found evidence for significant age-specific genetic effects on behavior in their longitudinal sample of twins assessed from ages 3 to 12. Results from longitudinal studies across childhood and adulthood are likewise inconsistent. In the study of male twin pairs from the Vietnam Era Twin Registry, Lyons et al. (1995) did not find any evidence for new genetic effects on adult antisocial behavior that were not shared with genetic influences on adolescent antisocial behavior. In contrast, Jacobson et al. (2002) reported significant effects of new genetic factors on both adolescent and adult antisocial behavior in their sample of male and female twins.

Although these results may at first appear contradictory, it is possible that the demonstration of age-specific effects is related to significant biological and social changes that may moderate the expression of genetic differences that occur during a relatively short window of time. For example, Bartels et al. (2004) found that the strongest evidence for age-specific genetic influence on antisocial behavior occurred sometime between the age 3 and age 7 assessments. It is possible that the presence of new genetic influence at age 7 was related to the marked developmental, social, and biological changes that occur between the ages of 3 and 6. Because the van den Oord and Rowe (1997) study combined the ages of 4–7 into a single assessment, they may have missed the critical period in which new genetic influences are expressed. Likewise, Jacobson et al. (2002) speculated that the presence of new genetic influence on adolescent antisocial behavior may be related to pubertal processes that "trigger" the expression of genetic influence. They supported this hypothesis by noting 1) that the presence of new genetic effects appeared later among males than females and 2) that although the heritability of child antisocial behavior was greater among females than among males, by middle adolescence and adulthood, the males had "caught up" to the females. Lyons et al. (1995), in their study, assessed antisocial behavior with only two distinct time periods, using a cutoff point of age 15. Thus, the measure of "adult" antisocial traits in this study included behaviors during middle and late adolescence, as well as adult behaviors. This choice of cutoff may have obscured any potential age-related changes.

Sources of Heterogeneity of Results Across Studies

Rater Effects

One of the most important factors to consider when comparing estimates of heritability at different ages *across studies* is that of potential *rater effects.* As can be seen in the review presented in the first part of this chapter, studies of antisocial behavior in early childhood typically find high estimates of heritability compared with studies of adolescent antisocial behavior, in which genetic influence is less certain. However, virtually all published studies of early childhood rely on ratings from others (typically parental ratings), whereas many of the studies of adolescent antisocial behavior rely on self-report. If the heritability of antisocial behavior varies systematically across reporter, biases due to rater effects could explain this particular pattern of results.

It has long been known that there are only modest correlations of reports of antisocial behavior across raters. Because of these relatively low levels of agreement across raters, it is difficult to know which person's view represents the most "accurate" perception of antisocial behavior. Agreement among parents and children regarding children's own behaviors is particularly poor. Possible explanations for this lack of agreement include the following:

1. *Differences among parents and children in interpreting and understanding the conceptualization of behaviors that are being assessed.* This is especially true for studies of young children, who may lack the cognitive capacity to understand the questions.
2. *Differences in response bias, in which parents or children may be more or less likely to report certain behaviors.* For example, parents are more likely than their children to report symptoms of

child oppositional behavior and inattention (Edelbrock et al. 1986; Loeber et al. 1989).

3. *Differences in parental supervision.* Parents are not around their children 24 hours a day, especially during adolescence, when children spend considerable amounts of time in unsupervised settings. Thus, parents have the potential to underreport certain behaviors, especially behaviors such as problem behavior, which children may be reluctant to disclose to their parents.

Potential rater effects can be particularly problematic in studies of multiple siblings in the same family (e.g., twin studies) when the same rater (usually the mother) is reporting on the behavior of both twins. If the mother has her own particular reporting bias, this could artificially influence twin correlations for both MZ and DZ twins. Such influence would result in an estimate of shared environmental influence that is upwardly biased. On the other hand, it has been suggested that mothers of MZ twins are more likely than mothers of DZ twins to view their twins as more similar (a violation of the equal environments assumption), or conversely, that mothers of DZ twins are more likely than mothers of MZ twins to rate the behavior of their twins more differently (a sibling contrast effect). These types of biases would result in artificially lower correlations for DZ twins compared with those for MZ twins, which would in turn result in heritability estimates that are upwardly biased.

Cross-sectional comparisons of results using different raters of antisocial behavior do sometimes yield higher estimates of both heritability and shared environmental influences for parental reports compared with other ratings, such as self-report (L. Baker, A. Raine, D. Lozano, manuscript in preparation, 2005; Simonoff et al. 1998). However, the only way to assess whether these higher heritabilities are due to parental bias or to different views of antisocial behavior is to conduct multivariate behavioral genetic models using data from multiple raters simultaneously. For example, Simonoff et al. (1995) obtained mother, father, and child reports of disruptive behaviors from families with adolescent male-male twin pairs. Results for questionnaire data revealed significant effects of a shared parental view. That is, mothers and fathers had higher levels of agreement with each other than either parent had with the children. This lends support to the hypothesis that part of the disagreement between parents and their children is due to situational specificity (i.e., parents do not see all of their children's behaviors, and children may behave quite differently at home than they do with their friends).

When these data were analyzed separately across rater, there was evidence for greater influence of shared environmental factors for mother and father reports (.42–.58) compared with child self-report (.34), although, interestingly, there was little difference in estimates of heritability across rater (.23–.34). When shared parental view was taken into account, estimates of shared environmental influence on the underlying latent phenotype were similar to those obtained through individual child self-report. Thus, although this study cannot determine whose viewpoint on behavior is "correct," it does provide evidence that studies of adolescents based on parental report may overestimate shared environmental influences.

Heterogeneity of Antisocial Behavior

So far, this chapter has focused on estimates of genetic and environmental influences on the development of antisocial behavior while assuming that antisocial behavior is a homogeneous phenomenon. However, during the past few decades, there has been increased recognition that antisocial behavior may, in fact, represent a heterogeneous phenomenon, with a variety of distinct causes and consequences.

Although use of behavioral genetic strategies to assess potential heterogeneity in antisocial behavior is a relatively new approach, two aspects of heterogeneity have received attention in behavioral genetic designs: 1) heterogeneity as defined by different *developmental trajectories* and 2) heterogeneity based on *comorbidity with other behaviors.*

Developmental Typologies of Antisocial Behavior

In a seminal article, Robins (1978) compared life-course patterns of antisocial behavior from four large, longitudinal, population-based studies. Consistent across all studies were two seemingly paradoxical findings: 1) most adults with ASPD had a history of childhood or adolescent conduct disorder, indicating substantial continuity of antisocial behavior across the life course; and 2) the majority of individuals with conduct disorder did not go on to become antisocial adults, suggesting some discontinuity to antisocial behavior (Robins 1978).

Results from the Cambridge Study of Delinquency among a single-birth cohort in the United Kingdom revealed similar patterns: delinquent behavior during adolescence was normative in this sample, with upward of 70% of male adolescents admitting to participating in at least one delinquent activity (West and Farrington 1973). However, the majority of adult criminal offenses were committed by the same 5%–6% of individuals (Farrington 1995). Finally, more recent examinations of sex differences in rates of antisocial or delinquent behavior have found that males outnumber females in various aspects of adult antisocial behavior (including criminal offenses and rates of adult ASPD) by a magnitude of 5–10 males to every 1 female, whereas the sex ratio for adolescent-onset antisocial behavior is more equal (approximately 1.5:1) (Moffitt and Caspi 2001). Taken together, the results from these studies suggest that the risk factors that influence transitory, adolescent-based antisocial behavior may differ from those that influence long-term, life-course persistent antisocial behavior.

Moffitt's (1993) theory of *life-course persistent* (LCP) versus *adolescent-limited* (AL) delinquency has been especially influential in current research on the development and heterogeneity of antisocial behavior. Moffitt emphasizes differences in timing, continuity, frequency, and severity of antisocial behavior across these two primary groups, and also points to different biological, psychological, and social mechanisms. In brief, *AL delinquency* is defined by transient antisocial behavior, with an onset generally in adolescence, that is less frequent and consists of more benign antisocial behaviors. In contrast, *LCP delinquency* is characterized by earlier onset of antisocial behavior, a wider variety of antisocial behaviors, higher rates of severe antisocial behavior (such as aggressive behavior), and more likelihood that the antisocial behavior will continue into adulthood (Moffitt 1993).

Recent research using longitudinal studies has also confirmed that LCP and AL delinquents can be differentiated on the basis of a number of social factors, including psychosocial risk composites comprising factors such as maternal depression, maternal life stress, low socioeconomic status (SES), single parenthood, home environment, and parental treatment (Aguilar et al. 2000); frequency of family transitions and disrupted family processes (e.g., Patterson et al. 1998); and inadequate parenting practices (Moffitt and Caspi 2001). In addition, accumulating evidence suggests that personality and temperamental factors—such as early childhood hyperactivity, fighting, and "difficulty" (Moffitt and Caspi 2001); lack of control (Henry et al. 1996); high impulsivity combined with low reward dependence (Tremblay et al. 1994); and lower cognitive ability (Donnellan et al. 2000)—may differentiate early-onset and later-onset delinquency. Overall, this body of research suggests that LCP and AL delinquents represent two distinct groups of individuals. Because behavioral genetic research concentrates on the underlying genetic and environmental influences on variation in human behavior and characteristics, genetically informative studies can be a useful tool for testing whether different groups of individuals have different genetic and environmental etiologies for the "same" phenotype.

In a 1989 review article on the genetics of aggressive behavior, DiLalla and Gottesman, like Moffitt, proposed that typologies based on different life-course patterns of antisocial behavior should yield different estimates of genetic and environmental influences. They predicted that AL antisocial behavior (individuals with such behavior were defined in their article as "transitory antisocials") should show the strongest influence of environment, particularly environments that are shared across children in the same family, such as community or neighborhood characteristics, family characteristics such as social class or education level, shared parental treatments, and shared peer influences. In contrast, they predicted that LCP antisocial behavior (individuals with such behavior were defined as "continuous antisocials") should show the strongest genetic influence (i.e., the highest heritabilities).

In this chapter, I have already reviewed a number of findings that may support the idea of genetic heterogeneity of antisocial behavior. The fact that longitudinal and quasi-longitudinal studies strongly indicate that genetic factors influence the continuity of antisocial behavior across childhood, adolescence, and adulthood may suggest that life-course patterns of antisocial behavior are genetically influenced. Likewise, the repeated findings of higher heritability for adult versus adolescent antisocial behavior might indicate that persistent patterns of antisocial behavior are more strongly influenced by genetic factors than are transient patterns of behavior. Finally, the increasing evidence for a higher heritability of aggressive versus nonaggressive antisocial behavior may also be taken as suggestive of a higher heritability among individuals with LCP patterns of antisocial behavior, who typically show more aggressive patterns of behavior than do individuals with AL patterns of antisocial behavior.

Nevertheless, although these studies offer indirect support for the hypothesis of differential genetic and environmental influence on different life-course patterns of antisocial behavior, they do not test this hypothesis directly. Predictions pertaining to different genetic and environmental etiologies of LCP and AL individuals require some type of *person-centered analyses* that focus on group differences in the relative influence of genetic and environmental factors on individual differences in antisocial behavior. To date, there are two studies that have revealed higher heritability of antisocial behavior among individuals with LCP patterns of antisocial behavior. Using a sample of 147 twin boys, ages 10 to 12 years, Taylor et al. (2000) tested the hypothesis that genetic influence on antisocial behavior would be greatest among "early starters" than among "late starters" or nondelinquents. They found higher rates of antisocial behavior among identical (i.e., monozygotic, or MZ) co-twins of early starters compared with fraternal (i.e., dizygotic, or DZ) co-twins of early starters, indicating genetic influence on antisocial behavior among early starters. In contrast, rates of antisocial behavior among co-twins of late starters were similar for MZ and DZ co-twins, indicating little or no genetic influence. Results were also replicated in an analysis of probandwise concordance rates, supporting the hypothesis of greater genetic influence on early-onset delinquency than on late-onset delinquency, and greater shared environmental influence on late-onset delinquency.

This first study focused on earlier age at onset as a potential indicator of the LCP pattern of antisocial behavior. One limitation of this study, however, is that the average age of the sample was quite young (mean age=11 years), so that subjects were not past the "risk-period" for normative adolescent delinquency, which typically peaks between ages 14 and 16. The second study, therefore, used data from adult twins from the Virginia Twin Registry to investigate whether the heritability of adolescent conduct-disordered behavior would be higher among individuals who *persisted* in their antisocial behavior during adulthood than among individuals who were not antisocial during adulthood (K.C. Jacobson, M.Neale, C.A. Prescott, et al., manuscript under review, 2005). Results of this study (Figure 6–3) confirmed the hypothesis that the heritability of adolescent conduct-disordered behavior was higher among individuals who were antisocial during adulthood as well, compared with individuals who were not antisocial during adulthood; conversely, shared environmental influences were significant only in the non-antisocial adult group. To the extent that persistence of antisocial behavior into adulthood represents a LCP pattern of behavior, these results are consistent with the hypothesis that heritabilities of LCP patterns of behavior are higher than those for AL antisocial behavior.

One important implication of the results from these studies is that the aforementioned conclusions concerning age-related changes in genetic influence on antisocial behavior may be overstated. In previous reviews and meta-analyses (e.g., Miles and Carey 1997), the aggregate heritability of antisocial behavior was estimated at approximately .20 among adolescents and .40–.50 among adults, suggesting modest genetic influence on antisocial behavior in adolescence and moderate genetic influence on antisocial behavior among adults. Results from the Jacobson et al. study (K.C. Jacobson et al., manuscript under review, 2005) indicate that moderately high levels of heritability for adolescent antisocial behavior do exist (.40), but only among specific subgroups of the population (i.e., individuals with LCP patterns of behavior). Interestingly, the estimate of heritability among the non-antisocial adult group (.20) was identical to the estimate of heritability of adolescent antisocial behavior in the Miles and Carey (1997) meta-analysis.

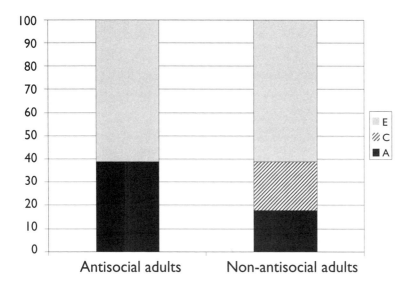

Figure 6–3. Genetic and environmental influences on adolescent conduct disorder.

A=additive genetic influence; C=shared environmental influence; E = nonshared environmental influence.

Moreover, results from these two studies of developmental heterogeneity may help to explain the somewhat counter-intuitive pattern of results from the studies of children, adolescents, and adults—namely, that the heritabilities of antisocial behavior in both child and adult samples are higher than the heritabilities obtained with adolescent samples. To the extent that early childhood problem behavior and continuation of antisocial behavior into adulthood are both manifestations of LCP patterns of behavior, this inverted U-shaped pattern of heritability is to be expected.

Patterns of Comorbidity With Antisocial Behavior

Psychiatrists and psychologists have recognized that comorbidity among psychiatric disorders is the norm, not the exception. In particular, conduct disorder is often comorbid with oppositional defiant disorder, ADHD, and substance use during adolescence, and ASPD is often comorbid with alcohol and drug disorders.

Moreover, there is considerable evidence from family, twin, and adoption studies that comorbidity in externalizing disorders is due to, at least in part, an overlap of common genetic factors (e.g., Eaves et al. 2000; Pickens et al. 1989; Schmitz and Mrazek 2001; Slutske et al. 1998; True et al. 1999). Of particular interest is the question of whether patterns of comorbidity can be used as a method for defining subtypes of antisocial behavior. Using latent class analysis in a sample of adolescent twins, Silberg et al. (1996a) found differences in genetic and environmental influences on different subtypes of antisocial behavior. Of most relevance are the results that variance in "pure" conduct-disordered behavior was largely due to shared environmental influences, whereas variation in comorbid conduct-disordered behavior was largely genetic in origin. These results again support the hypothesis that more extreme, pathological antisocial behavior is more strongly influenced by genetic factors than is "normative" adolescent antisocial behavior.

Gene × Environment Interactions (G×E) in the Study of Antisocial Behavior

In this chapter, I have largely focused on the additive roles of genetic and environmental factors in the etiology of delinquent, antisocial, aggressive, and criminal behavior. In other words, many traditional twin and adoption models assume that genetic and environmental factors have unique and independent effects on variation in behavior. However, there is a growing consensus that genetic and environmental influences on variation in antisocial behavior may not operate in such a straightforward, linear fashion and that studies that attempt to identify the *independent* effects of genetic and environmental factors may mask the true complexity of organism-environment *interaction.*

Promising directions for research on aggressive and criminal behavior can be found in models that emphasize the *joint* influences of both environment and biology. Examples of such models are the biosocial perspective (e.g., Raine et al. 1997a) and the diathesis stress model currently used in behavioral genetic research on psychopathology (including aggressive behaviors) (e.g., Cadoret et al. 1995; Kendler and Eaves 1986). What is particularly novel about these approaches is that in addition to acknowledging that biology, genes, and environments may contribute independently to development of criminality, both models emphasize the point that these factors may also interact with one another to influence behavior. In particular, it is thought that a genetic "liability" toward aggressive and criminal behavior may be expressed only in a given environment—most often a harsh rearing environment.

For example, Raine et al. (1997b) reported that birth complications interacted with early maternal rejection to predict adult violence. Specifically, adult violent offenders were more likely to have experienced both birth complications and early maternal rejection than just one of these risk factors. The interactive effect of birth complications and early maternal rejection was especially strong in predicting the onset of violence before age 18 (Raine et al. 1997b). Interestingly, the authors found that this interaction effect did not generalize to nonviolent criminal offenses. Similar results were reported in a large birth cohort sample from Sweden (Hodgins et al. 2001).

Recently, studies have examined community- and family-level risk factors as potential moderators of biological or genetic indices of vulnerability to antisocial behavior. Results from the Pittsburgh Youth Study found that the relationship between impulsivity and juvenile offending was stronger for boys in poorer neighborhood (Lynam et al. 2000). In addition, poorer environments were not associated with higher levels of juvenile offending among nonimpulsive boys, suggesting that environmental risk has a significant effect on offending only among individuals with potentially predisposing personality characteristics. What is particularly impressive about this study is that the initial, cross-sectional results from 13-year-old males were replicated at age 17 with a longitudinal design.

Using data from male American veterans, Dabbs and Morris (1990) reported that higher levels of testosterone predicted adult deviance and retrospective reports of childhood delinquency only among males from a low SES background. Among adolescents from higher SES backgrounds, testosterone was not related to childhood or adult deviance. Likewise, a different study using the same sample found an interaction effect between testosterone levels and a measure of social integration (defined by factors such as educational attainment, organizational ties, job stability, and marriage) for adult deviance (Booth and Osgood 1993). Specifically, the difference in adult deviance associated with low, medium, and high levels of testosterone was greatest when participants reported low levels of social integration. When social integration was high, there was virtually no relationship between level of testosterone and adult deviance.

There is also evidence from behavioral genetic studies for genetic × environmental interactions (G×E) in the development of antisocial behavior. For example, Cadoret and colleagues found evidence for an "environmental trigger" in their Iowa adoption study of aggressivity and conduct disorders (Cadoret et al. 1995, 1997). In this study, biological risk, defined as having a biological parent with ASPD, interacted with adverse adoptive home environments (defined by factors such as psychopathology, drug abuse, and divorce or separation in the adoptive family) to predict diagnoses of child and adolescent aggressivity and conduct disorder. For example, Figure 6–4 shows the relationship between number of adverse home environmental factors and number of adolescent aggressivity symptoms for adoptees with and without a biological parent with ASPD. Among adoptees without a biological parent with ASPD, there was no relationship between number of adverse adoptive home environment factors and number of aggressivity symptoms. In contrast, among adoptees with a biological parent diagnosed with ASP, the number of aggressivity symptoms increased with the number of adverse adoptive home environmental factors. Cadoret et al. (1997) also reported that specific environmental conditions, such as conflict with the adoptive mother and father, interacted with biological predisposition to predict adolescent aggressive behavior.

Finally, one of the first published studies of *measured GxE* for a complex behavioral phenotype focused on the interaction between a genotype that codes for monoamine oxidase–A (MAO-A) activity and the environmental risk of child maltreatment as a possible explanation for why some individuals from abusive homes do not grow up to be violent themselves (Caspi et al. 2002).

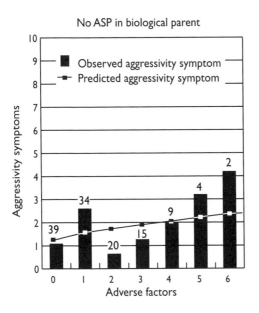

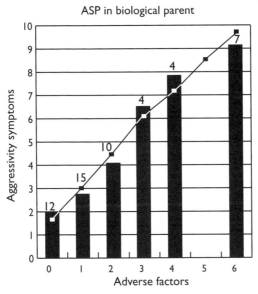

Figure 6–4. Interaction between biological risk and adverse environmental experiences.

Numbers over bars indicate observations. ASP=antisocial personality.

Source. Reprinted from Cadoret RJ, Leve LD, Devor E: "Genetics of Aggressive and Violent Behavior." *Psychiatric Clinics of North America* 20:301–322, 1997. Used with permission.

The results from this study, which used a longitudinal sample of males assessed from childhood to adulthood, indicate that a polymorphism that codes for high MAO-A activity mitigated the adverse effects of child maltreatment on a variety of antisocial behavior outcomes, including conduct disorder, adult antisocial behavior, and convictions for violent offenses. Remarkably, a significant interaction with this same polymorphism and child maltreatment was recently replicated in the Virginia Adolescent Behavioral Development Study for maternal ratings of conduct-disordered behavior (Foley et al. 2004). In both studies, although there was a significant main effect of the environmental risk factor (child maltreatment), there was no main effect of genotype. Thus, molecular genetic studies that fail to consider the potential moderating effects of the environment may miss potentially significant genetic influences on antisocial behavior.

Conclusion

In this chapter, I have reviewed the basic behavioral genetic literature on the development of antisocial behavior, focusing particularly on potential age-related changes in the expression of genetic influence (i.e., changes in heritability). Three potential explanations were given to explain the differences across studies in the magnitude of genetic influence on antisocial behavior at different ages: 1) a potential rater bias effect, 2) actual developmental changes due to relevant social and biological factors that either trigger or suppress genetic influence, and 3) heterogeneity masking as developmental change. In addition, I focused on the potential for the complex interplay between genes and environment to be an important process in the development of antisocial behavior. From a clinical standpoint, it seems clear that both genetic and environmental factors play an important role in the development of antisocial behavior. Genetic factors appear to be particularly important for the development of more severe, life-course persistent patterns of antisocial behavior. Nevertheless, there is increasing evidence that genetic risk, or family history of antisocial behavior, may be insufficient, in and of itself, as a direct causal factor in the development of problem behavior. Instead, adverse environmental experiences may trigger latent genetic liability to antisocial behavior. This hypothesis has important implications for treating individuals who exhibit antisocial behavior, as it suggests that modifications to the environment may be an effective means of suppressing these latent liabilities.

References

Achenbach TM, Edelbrock CS: The Child Behavior Profile, II: boys aged 12–16 and girls aged 6–11 and 12–16. J Consult Clin Psychol 47:223–233, 1979

Aguilar B, Sroufe LA, Egeland B, et al: Distinguishing the early-onset/persistent and adolescence-onset antisocial behavior types: from birth to 16 years. Dev Psychopathol 12:109–132, 2000

American Psychiatric Association: Diagnostic and Statistical Manual of Mental Disorders, 3rd Edition, Revised. Washington, DC, American Psychiatric Association, 1987

American Psychiatric Association: Diagnostic and Statistical Manual of Mental Disorders, 4th Edition. Washington, DC, American Psychiatric Association, 1994

American Psychiatric Association: Diagnostic and Statistical Manual of Mental Disorders, 4th Edition, Text Revision. Washington, DC, American Psychiatric Association, 2000

Arsenault L, Moffitt TE, Caspi A, et al: Strong genetic effects on cross-situational antisocial behaviour among 5-year-old children according to mothers, teachers, examiner-observers, and twins' self-reports. J Child Psychol Psychiatry 44:832–848, 2003

Bartels M, van den Oord EJCG, Hudziak JJ, et al: Genetic and environmental mechanisms underlying stability and change in problem behaviors at ages 3, 7, 10, and 12. Dev Psychol 40:852–867, 2004

Booth A, Osgood DW: The influence of testosterone on deviance in adulthood: assessing and explaining the relationship. Criminology 31:93–117, 1993

Brennan PA, Mednick SA: Genetic perspectives on crime. Acta Psychiatr Scand Suppl 370:19–26, 1993

Cadoret RJ: Psychopathology in adopted-away offspring of biologic parents with antisocial behavior. Arch Gen Psychiatry 35:176–184, 1978

Cadoret RJ, Yates WR, Troughton E, et al: Genetic-environmental interaction in the genesis of aggressivity and conduct disorders. Arch Gen Psychiatry 52:916–924, 1995

Cadoret RJ, Leve LD, Devor E: Genetics of aggressive and violent behavior. Psychiatr Clin North Am 20:301–322, 1997

Caspi A, McClay J, Moffitt TE, et al: Role of genotype in the cycle of violence in maltreated children. Science 297:851–854, 2002

Cloninger CR, Gottesman II: Genetic and environmental factors in antisocial behavior disorder, in The Causes of Crime: New Biological Approaches. Edited by Mednick SA, Moffitt TE, Stack SA. Cambridge, England, Cambridge University Press, 1997, pp 92–109

Costello EJ, Edelbrock CS, Costello AJ: Validity of the NIMH Diagnostic Interview Schedule for Children: a comparison between psychiatric and pediatric referrals. J Abnorm Child Psychol 13:579–595, 1985

Dabbs JM Jr, Morris R: Testosterone, social class, and antisocial behavior in a sample of 4,462 men. Psychol Sci 1:209-211, 1990

Deater-Deckard K, Plomin R: An adoption study of teacher and parent reports of externalizing behavior problems in middle childhood. Child Dev 70:144–154, 1999

DiLalla LF, Gottesman II: Heterogeneity of causes for delinquency and criminality: lifespan perspectives. Dev Psychopathol 1:339–349, 1989

Donnellan MB, Ge X, Wenk E: Cognitive abilities in adolescent-limited and life-course-persistent criminal offenders. J Abnorm Psychol 109: 396–402, 2000

Eaves LJ, Silberg JL, Meyer JM, et al: Genetics and developmental psychopathology, 2: the main effects of genes and environment on behavioral problems in the Virginia Twin Study of Adolescent Behavioral Development. J Child Psychol Psychiatry 38:965–980, 1997

Eaves LJ, Rutter M, Silberg JL, et al: Genetic and environmental causes of covariation in interview assessments of disruptive behavior in child and adolescent twins. Behav Genet 30:321–334, 2000

Edelbrock CS, Costello AM, Dulcan MK, et al: Parent-child agreement on child psychiatric symptoms assessed via structured interview. J Child Psychol Psychiatry 27:181–190, 1986

Edelbrock CS, Rende R, Plomin R, et al: A twin study of competence and problem behavior in childhood and early adolescence. J Child Psychol Psychiatry 56:775–785, 1995

Eley TC, Lichtenstein P, Stevenson J: Sex differences in the etiology of aggressive and nonaggressive antisocial behavior: results from two twin studies. Child Dev 70:155–168, 1999

Eley TC, Lichtenstein P, Moffit TE: A longitudinal behavioral genetic analysis of the etiology of aggressive and nonaggressive antisocial behavior. Dev Psychopathol 15:383–402, 2003

Faraone SV, Biederman J, Monuteaux MC: Attention-deficit disorder and conduct disorder in girls: evidence for a familial subtype. Biol Psychiatry 48:21–29, 2000

Farrington DP: The Twelfth Jack Tizard Memorial Lecture: The development of offending and antisocial behaviour from childhood: key findings from the Cambridge Study in Delinquent Development. J Child Psychol Psychiatry 36:929–964, 1995

Foley DL, Eaves LJ, Wormley B, et al: Childhood adversity, monoamine oxidase A, genotype, and risk for conduct disorder. Arch Gen Psychiatry 61:738–741, 2004

Ghodsian-Carpey J, Baker LA: Genetic and environmental influences on aggression in 4- to 7-year-old twins. Aggress Behav 13:173–186, 1987

Gjone H, Stevenson J: A longitudinal twin study of temperament and behavior problems: common genetic or environmental influences? J Am Acad Child Adolesc Psychiatry 36:1448–1456, 1997

Henry B, Caspi A, Moffitt T, et al: Temperamental and familial predictors of violent and nonviolent criminal convictions: age 3 to age 18. Dev Psychol 32:614–623, 1996

Hodgins S, Kratzer L, McNeil TF: Obstetric complications, parenting, and risk of criminal behavior. Arch Gen Psychiatry 58:746–752, 2001

Jacobson KC, Prescott CA, Kendler KS: Sex differences in genetic and environmental influences on antisocial behavior from childhood to adulthood. Dev Psychopathol 14:395–416, 2002

Kendler KS, Eaves LJ: Models for the joint effect of genotype and environment on liability to psychiatric illness. Am J Psychiatry 143:279–289, 1986

Loeber R, Hay D: Key issues in development of aggression and violence from childhood to early adulthood. Ann Rev Psychol 48:371–410, 1991

Loeber R, Green SM, Lahey BB, et al: Optimal informants on childhood disruptive behaviors. Dev Psychopathol 1:317–337, 1989

Lynam DR: Pursuing the psychopath: capturing the fledgling psychopath in a nomological net. J Abnorm Psychol 106:425–438, 1997

Lynam DR, Caspi A, Moffitt TE, et al: The interaction between impulsivity and neighborhood context on offending: the effects of impulsivity are stronger in poorer neighborhoods. J Abnorm Psychol 109:563–574, 2000

Lyons MJ, True WR, Eisen SA, et al: Differential heritability of adult and juvenile antisocial traits. Arch Gen Psychiatry 52:906–915, 1995

Mannuzza S, Klein RG, Konig PH, et al: Hyperactive boys almost grown up, IV: criminality and its relationship to psychiatric status. Arch Gen Psychiatry 46:1073–1079, 1989

Mednick SA, Gabrielli WF Jr., Hutchings B: Genetic influences in criminal convictions: evidence from an adoption cohort. Science 224:891–894, 1984

Miles DR, Carey G: Genetic and environmental architecture of human aggression. J Pers Soc Psychol 72:207–217, 1997

Moffitt T: Adolescence-limited and life-course-persistent antisocial behavior: a developmental taxonomy. Psychol Rev 100:674–701, 1993

Moffitt T, Caspi A: Childhood predictors differentiate life-course persistent and adolescence-limited antisocial pathways among males and females. Dev Psychopathol 13:355–375, 2001

Neiderhiser JM, Reiss D, Hetherington EM: Genetically informative designs for distinguishing pathways during adolescence: responsible and antisocial behavior. Dev Psychopathol 8:779–791, 1996

O'Connor TG, Neiderhiser JM, Reiss D, et al: Genetic contributions to continuity, change, and co-occurrence of antisocial and depressive symptoms in adolescence. J Child Psychol Psychiatry 39:323–336, 1998

Patterson GR, Forgatch MS, Yoerger KL, et al: Variables that initiate and maintain an early-onset trajectory for juvenile offending. Dev Psychopathol 10:531–547, 1998

Pickens RW, Svikis DS, McGue M, et al: Common genetic mechanisms in alcohol drug and mental disorder comorbidity. Drug Alcohol Depend 39:129–138, 1989

Plomin R: Development, Genetics, and Psychology. Hillsdale, NJ, Erlbaum, 1986

Raine A, Brennan P, Farrington DP: Biosocial bases of violence: conceptual and theoretical issues, in Biosocial Bases of Violence. Edited by Raine A, Brennan P, Farrington DP, et al. New York, Plenum, 1997a, pp 1–21

Raine A, Brennan P, Mednick SA: Interaction between birth complications and early maternal rejection in predisposing individuals to adult violence: specificity to serious, early-onset violence. Am J Psychiatry 154:1265–1271, 1997b

Rhee SH, Waldman ID: Genetic and environmental influences on antisocial behavior: a meta-analysis of twin and adoption studies. Psychol Bull 128:490–529, 2002

Robins LN: Sturdy childhood predictors of adult antisocial behaviour: replications from longitudinal studies. Psychol Med 8:611–622, 1978

Rowe DC: A biometrical analysis of perceptions of family environment: a study of twin and singleton sibling kinships. Child Dev 54:416–423, 1983

Satterfield JH, Hoppe CM, Schell AM: A prospective study of delinquency in 110 adolescent boys with attention deficit disorder and 88 normal adolescent boys. Am J Psychiatry 139:795–798, 1982

Schmitz S, Mrazek DA: Genetic and environmental influences on the associations between attention problems and other problem behaviors. Twin Research 4:453–458, 2001

Schmitz S, Cherny SS, Fulker DW, et al: Genetic and environmental influences on early childhood behavior. Behav Genet 24:25–34, 1994

Silberg JL, Meyer J, Pickles A, et al: Heterogeneity among juvenile antisocial behaviours: findings from the Virginia Twin Study of Adolescent Behavioral Development, in Genetics of Criminal and Antisocial Behaviour (Ciba Foundation Symposium 194). Chichester, England, Wiley, 1996a, pp 76–92

Silberg J, Rutter M, Meyer J, et al: Genetic and environmental influences on the covariation between hyperactivity and conduct disturbance in juvenile twins. J Child Psychol Psychiatry 37:803–816, 1996b

Simonoff E, Pickles A, Hewitt J, et al: Multiple raters of disruptive child behavior: using a genetic strategy to examine shared views and bias. Behav Genet 25:311–326, 1995

Simonoff E, Pickles A, Meyer J, et al: Genetic and environmental influences on subtypes of conduct disorder behavior in boys. J Abnorm Child Psychol 26:495–509, 1998

Simonoff E, Eleander J, Holmshaw J, et al: Predictors of antisocial personality. Br J Psychol 184:118–127, 2004

Slutske WS: The genetics of antisocial behavior. Current Psychiatry Reports 3:158–162, 2001

Slutske WS, Heath AC, Dinwiddie SH, et al: Modeling genetic and environmental influences in the etiology of conduct disorder: a study of 2,682 adult twin pairs. J Abnorm Psychol 106:266–279, 1997

Slutske WS, Heath AC, Dinwiddie SH, et al: Common genetic risk factors for conduct disorder and alcohol dependence. J Abnorm Psychol 107:363–374, 1998

Stattin H, Magnusson D: The role of early aggressive behavior in the frequency, seriousness, and types of later crimes. J Consult Clin Psychol 57:710–718, 1989

Taylor J, Iacono WG, McGue M: Evidence for a genetic etiology of early-onset delinquency. J Abnorm Psychol 109:634–643, 2000

Thapar A, McGuffin P: A twin study of antisocial and neurotic symptoms in childhood. Psychol Med 26:1111–1118, 1996

Tremblay RE, Pihl RO, Vitaro F, et al: Predicting early onset of male antisocial behavior from preschool behavior. Arch Gen Psychiatry 51:732–739, 1994

True WR, Heath AC, Scherrer JF, et al: Interrelationship of genetic and environmental influences on conduct disorder and alcohol and marijuana dependence symptoms. Am J Med Genet 88:391–397, 1999

van den Oord EJC, Rowe DC: Continuity and change in children's social maladjustment: a developmental behavior genetic study. Dev Psychol 33:319–322, 1997

van den Oord EJ, Velhurst FC, Boomsma DI: A genetic study of maternal and paternal ratings of problem behaviors in 3-year-old twins. J Abnorm Psychol 105:349–357, 1996

West DJ, Farrington DP: Who Becomes Delinquent? Second Report of the Cambridge Study in Delinquent Development. Oxford, England, Crane, Russak, 1973

Index

*Page numbers printed in **boldface** type refer to tables or figures.*

Generalized anxiety disorder
(GAD), 147–149
family studies, 147–148
twin studies, 148–149
Genetic epidemiological studies.
See Epidemiological studies
Genetic risk factors, 2, 10–11,
25–27
Genetic variants (markers), 5
Genome
scan, 51
screen data, 127–128
Genotype-environment
correlation (rGE), 29, 34,
75–79, **76–77**
Genotype × environment
interaction (G×E), 29, 72–73,
74–75
in antisocial behavior studies,
222–226, **225**
in schizophrenia, 101
G×E. *See* Genotype × environment
interaction (G×E)

Haplotypes, 5, 57, 112
Headaches, 145
Heritability, 2, 6, 7
Heterogeneity, 27
sources of antisocial behavior,
214–222
Heterozygosity, 113
Holistic approach, 19
Hypothetico-deductive method,
31

Illicit substances abuse and
dependence, 184–186
Imprinting, 27
Inflammatory bowel disease, 129
Influences on substance use
disorders, 187–192

Insertions, 57
Integration, 12–13

Late childhood, antisocial
behavior, 200–206
Latent variables, 33, 63
for twin resemblance, **42,** 42–46
Life-course persistent
delinquency (LCP), 217–221
Linear Structural Relations
(LISREL), 63
Linkage disequilibrium, 55, 111
Linkage studies, 50–55, 62–63.
See also Molecular genetic
studies
chromosomes, 115–126, **119**
schizophrenia, 103–110,
105–106, 108, 112–128
substance use disorders,
178–179, 182–183
LISREL. *See* Linear Structural
Relations (LISREL)
Locus, 4–5, 99
LOD scores, 104–107. 123, 124,
125, 127, 145–146, 152, 179
Longitudinal genetic studies, 68,
144, 209–210

Major depressive disorder
(MDD), 148
Markers, 5, 50–63
association studies, 55–56
linkage studies, 51–55
nomenclature for, 114
sequence variation, 56–61
types, 113–115
MDD. *See* Major depressive
disorder (MDD)
Measured environment, 79
Meiosis, 8, 104
Mendel, Gregor, 22–23

Path models, 30–87, **35, 64, 65.**
 See also Structural equation
   modeling
 adoption studies, 47–50
 developmental process, 67–72
 endophenotypes, 37–39, **38**
 familial resemblance, 39–47
 G×E interaction, 72–73, **74–75**
 linkage and association,
   50–63
 multiple variables, 63–67
 parental effects, 79–83, **80**
 quantitative trait loci (QTLs),
   36–37
 rGE correlation, 75–79, **76–77**
 statistics, 83–87
 for substance use disorders,
   188, 189
 twin resemblance, **42,** 42–46
Pathogenic variants, 5
PCR. *See* Polymerase chain
   reaction (PCR)
PD. *See* Panic disorder (PD)
Pedigree disequilibrium testing
   (PDT), 112
Persistence phenotype, 180
Phenotype
 genetic effects, 26
 path model, **35**
Phobias, 149–152
 family studies, 149–150, **151**
 molecular genetic studies,
   150–152
 twin studies, 150
Pleiotropy, 27
Polygenic theory of continuous
   variation, 23
Polymerase chain reaction (PCR),
   59–60
Polymorphisms, 56–61, **58**
 kinds of, 57

Population attributable risk
   (PAR), 116
Population stratification, 55–56,
   111
Posttraumatic stress disorder
   (PTSD), 157–159
 family studies, 157
 molecular genetic studies, 158
 twin studies, 157–158
POT. *See* Parents of twins (POT)
Power calculations, 84–87, **86**
PPD. *See* Paranoid personality
   disorder (PPD)
PTSD. *See* Posttraumatic stress
   disorder (PTSD)

Quantitative trait loci (QTLs), 36–
   37

"Radical environmentalist"
Recombination, 104
Reductionist approach, 19
Reductive explanation, 7–8, 9
Replacement, 12
Replication, 128–129
Resemblance, twins, path model
   for, **42,** 42–47, **53, 54**
RGE. *See* Genotype-environment
   correlation (rGE)

Schizoaffective disorder, 102
Schizophrenia, 95–131
 analyses of genome screen
   data, 127–128
 association studies, 103, 111–
   112
 compared with Mendelian
   disorders, 107–110
 genetic epidemiology, 96–103
 linkage analysis, 103–110,
   105–106, 108